ENVIRONMENTAL FACTORS AND MALARIA TRANSMISSION RISK

To all families affected by malaria,
hope is on the horizon

Environmental Factors and Malaria Transmission Risk

Modelling the Risk in a Holoendemic Area of Burkina Faso

YAZOUMÉ YÉ
African Population and Health Research Centre, Kenya

OSMAN SANKOH
INDEPTH Network, Ghana

BOCAR KOUYATÉ
Centre National de Recherche et de Formation sur le Paludisme, Burkina Faso

RAINER SAUERBORN
University of Heidelberg, Germany

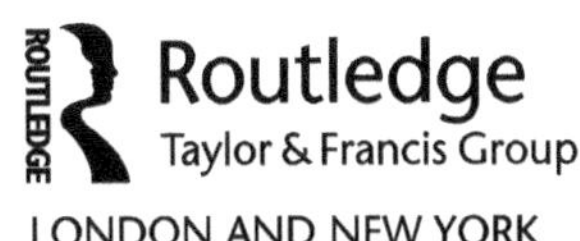

LONDON AND NEW YORK

First published 2008 by Ashgate Publishing

Reissued 2018 by Routledge
2 Park Square, Milton Park, Abingdon, Oxon OX14 4RN
711 Third Avenue, New York, NY 10017, USA

Routledge is an imprint of the Taylor & Francis Group, an informa business

First issued in paperback 2018

A Library of Congress record exists under LC control number: 2008030036

ISBN 13: 978-0-815-38882-1 (hbk)
ISBN 13: 978-1-138-61957-9 (pbk)
ISBN 13: 978-1-351-15900-5 (ebk)

Contents

List of Figures

List of Tables

List of Acronyms

An.	Anopheles
CCD	Cold Cloud Day
CDC-LT	Centres of Disease Control and prevention Light Trap
CRSN	Centre de Recherche en Santé de Nouna
DDT	Dichlorodiphenyl Trichloroethane
DSS	Demographic Surveillance Systems
EIR	Entomological Inoculation Rate
GIS	Geographical Information Systems
GPS	Global Positioning Systems
HBI	Human Blood Index
HBR	Human Biting Rate
HLC	Human Land Capture
LST	Land Surface Temperature
LTC	Light Trap Capture
MODIS	Moderate Resolution Imaging Spectroradiometer
NDVI	Normative Difference Vegetation Index
NOAA-AVHRR	National Oceanographic and Atmospheric Administration Advanced Very High Resolution Radiometer
NSM	Non Spatial Model
P. falciparum	*Plasmodium falciparum*
PSC	Pyrethrum Spray Capture
RH	Relative Humidity
RS	Remote Sensing
SPOT	Satellite pour l'Observation de la Terre
VC	Vectorial Capacity
VI	Vegetation Index
WHO	World Health Organization

Preface

Malaria although preventable remains a deadly disease and a serious public health problem worldwide and especially in developing countries. In Burkina Faso it accounts for about 20% of the under five mortality. The fifth Millennium Development Goal which is reducing infant mortality by two-thirds by the year 2015 can only be achieved if mortality caused by malaria is reduced. Among other strategies for reducing the malaria burden, the WHO recommends early detection and treatment among high-risk groups. To be effective this approach would need an early warning system (EWS) which allows the health care system to be well prepared and to allocate scarce resources effectively. Unfortunately, such a system is not available at the proper scale. This study, therefore, is filling this gap by developing a malaria transmission model at a local (district) scale using environmental factors. We set out to address the following research questions: i) To what extent does weather at the micro scale level affect malaria transmission among children under five (U5s) in a holoendemic area? and ii) Can malaria be predicted at local scale using weather parameters as a driving force?

The specific objectives were:

i. To assess the incidence of *P. falciparum* infection and clinical malaria among U5s in four different ecological settings in a holoendemic area, north-western Burkina Faso.
ii. To determine the effect of temperature, rainfall and relative humidity on *P. falciparum* infection risk among U5s in a holoendemic area.
iii. To determine the impact of temperature, rainfall on mosquitoes population dynamics in a holoendemic area.
iv. To assess the *P. falciparum* seasonal transmission pressure among U5s in a holoendemic area.
v. To develop and validate a dynamic, weather-based model of predicting malaria transmission risk.

To address these objectives we conducted a population-based cohort study. 867 children aged between 6 and 59 months were recruited through a random selection of their household from three villages (Goni, Cissé and Kodougou) and Nouna town. Interviewers followed these children for 12 months (01.12.2003–30.11.2004) over one dry and one rainy season for active parasite detection. The study started and ended with a cross-sectional survey. In addition, we assessed prospective exposure variables such as land cover, meteorological factors (temperature, rainfall, and relative humidity) and mosquito bites with ground-based data collection.

We have shown that *P. falciparum* infection incidence in the four sites is perennial with seasonal variation. The transmission peak is in the rainy season. Children in Goni and Kodougou have the highest incidence of *P. falciparum* infection. Nouna, a semi-urban site has the lowest. In the multivariate model using conventional logistic regression, only children in Kodougou have shown significant increase of odds of *P. falciparum* infection compared to those in Nouna. This difference was cancelled when, in a random effects model, we considered individual- and household-level variation. This suggests that given the same conditions (individual and household) the odds of *P. falciparum* infection are similar in all the sites.

P. falciparum infection among children is regulated by weather which impacts on the malaria vector population dynamic. Although all the individual weather parameters (with a lag of one month) have an impact on *P. falciparum* infection, mean temperature is the best predictor and the main driver.

Mosquito populations are mostly *Culex* species caught mainly in the urban site (Nouna). The most prominent specie among the malaria vectors was *Anopheles gambiae*. Temperature and rainfall regulated *Anopheles gambiae* population dynamics. Goni has the largest vector population because of its ecological setting.

The transmission pressure (EIR) is seasonal and varies significantly among sites. It was high in Goni, because of vector abundance. This has led to a high crude incidence of *P. falciparum* infection. Surprisingly, the transmission pressure was low in Kodougou despite its closeness to a perennial river.

We were able to develop and test a dynamic model of malaria transmission using the knowledge produced by this comprehensive time series data and the results provided by the different analyses. The dynamic model driven by temperature and rainfall successfully simulated seasonal vector abundance for each site. It also predicted successfully the monthly malaria incidence. However, the model needs to be tested for longer periods since the year in which the data was collected was not an average year for weather parameters.

Acknowledgments

The authors would like to express their gratitude to all the people who made this happen.

Special thanks go to Dr Moshe Hoshen for his scientific support in developing the malaria model. Despite his busy schedule he found time to spend two weeks on two separate occasions in Heidelberg, to work on the data. His scientific inputs in this book are invaluable. Many thanks to Dr Pitt Reitmaier for his support and scientific guidance.

Our gratitude goes to Prof. David Rogers from the University of Oxford for his thorough comments on the initial proposal for this work. They have helped greatly in tuning this project to the right wavelength.

Thanks to Prof. Pim Martens from the University of Maastricht and Prof. Dietz Klaus for their comments and suggestions at the preliminary stage of the proposal.

We are grateful to Dr Catherine Kyobutungi (African Population and Health Research Centre) and Dr Louis Valerie (University of Heidelberg) for their remarkable proofreading work and for the scientific comments and suggestions.

Many thanks to the (CRSN) team for their support in the data collection phase. The authors particularly want to thank the people who have directly contributed to the fieldwork for their remarkable work. They are:

Weather monitoring: Seraphin Simboro, who coordinated the fieldwork.

Parasitological team: Dr Boubacar Coulibaly, Issouf Traoré, Mohammed Diaby, Ibrahim Dissa Sory, Omer Kiénou, Dieudonné Zerbo.

Clinical team: Dr Florent Somé (RIP), Justin Tiendrebeogo.

Entomological team: Dr Ido Kolé, Seydou Ouedraogo, Francois D. Gonro, Thomas D. Dembélé, Hamidou Ouedraogo, Oumarou Ilboudo.

Data management: Alphonse Zagané, Cheik Bagagnan, Marie Rose Yelkouni, Sama Bienco.

We remain indebted to the study participants, including the children and their parents. Many thanks, from the depth of our hearts for their open collaboration, although the study was a burden for them.

This work was only possible because of the combined financial support from the German Research Council (DFG) – University of Heidelberg (within the framework of the Graduiertenkolleg 793) and the Union des Banques Suisse (UBS) Optimus Foundation. We will be forever grateful to these institutions.

Yazoumé Yé, Osman Sankoh, Bocar Kouyaté and Rainer Sauerborn

Chapter 1
Introduction

1.1 What is malaria? How is it transmitted?

1.1.1 Short history

The term "malaria", meaning "bad air" (*mal'aria*) in Italian was first used by Lancisi in 1717, who linked the recurrent fevers to the closeness of marshy and notoriously foul-smelling areas. In the fifth century BC, Hippocrates reported clinical details of malaria. In 1880, Laveran a French Army medical doctor, in Algeria, described the malaria parasite in humans and won the Nobel Prize for his work in 1907. Golgi identified and described the *Plasmodium vivax* and *malariae* in 1886 in Italy, while Cilli and Marchiafawa fully described the life cycle of *P. falciparum* in 1889. In 1897 Ronald Ross identified malaria oocysts in the gut wall of a female anopheline mosquito. This discovery clearly linked the parasite to the vector, and the theory of malaria transmission to humans by *Anopheles* species was accepted in 1898, resulting in a Nobel Prize in 1902 (Gilles and Warrel 1993).

1.1.2 Transmission cycle

Malaria is transmitted to humans by the female Anopheles mosquito, whose development is strongly dependent on the physical environment. The transmission cycle involves three major components (Figure 1.1), which are human (recipient), mosquito (vector), and environment (habitat), and can be subdivided into two subcycles: parasite cycle and mosquito cycle.

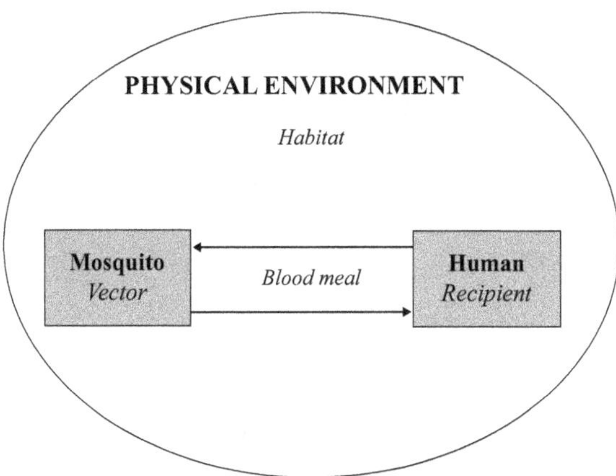

Figure 1.1 Malaria transmission cycle

1.1.2.1 Parasite cycle Four protozoan parasites are responsible for human malaria. They are *P. falciparum*, *P. vivax*, *P. ovale* and *P. malariae*. *P. falciparum* is the most virulent and life-threatening. The parasite development cycle involves the human and the vector hosts (Figure 1.2).

- In the human host
  The infected female mosquito *Anopheles* bites a person and injects saliva containing *Plasmodium* sporozoites into the bloodstream. The sporozoites enter the liver cells and grow to a schizont which multiplies (schizogony) and produces 2,000–4,000 merozoites. The merozoites will either infect other liver cells and repeat the cycle or pass into the blood and enter the erythrocyte (red blood cell) in the schizogonous cycle. The liver stage lasts from 6 to 16 days. An individual merozoite in a red blood cell will produce 6–24 merozoites. The cycle is repeated several times so the number of infected erythrocytes in the bloodstream increases enormously. The duration of the cycle is the duration between successive bouts of fever which correspond to rupture of the red blood cells (Gilles and Warrel 1993). A part of merozoites will stop multiplying and asexually transform into male and female gametocytes.

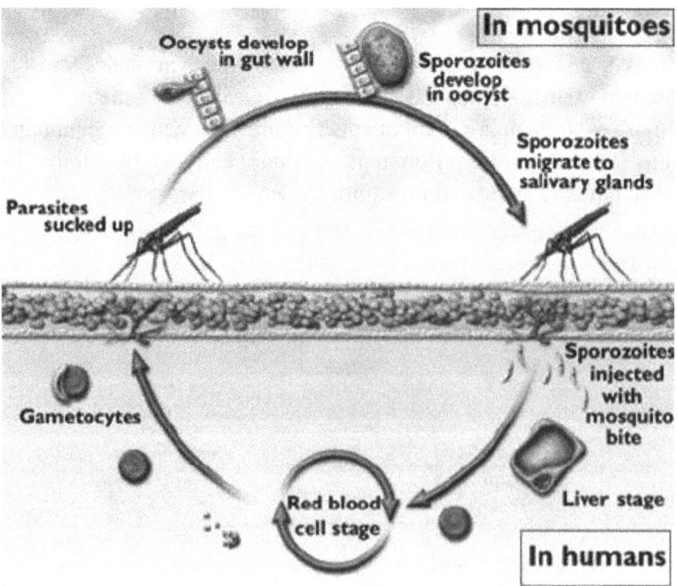

Figure 1.2 Malaria parasite cycle
(*Source*: www.traveldoctor.co.uk/ malaria.htm)

- In the vector host
  When a mosquito bites an infected person, it injects saliva and sucks up blood with the merozoites and gametocytes. The merozoites are digested in the mosquito's gut but the gametocytes survive. Female gametocytes transform into macrogametes (females gametes) and male ones into microgametes (male gametes). A macrogamete will be fertilised by exflagellation of microgametes to give a "zygote". The zygote develops into an ookinete over 12 to 48 hours and penetrates the wall of the midgut and becomes an oocyst. As the oocyst grows its contents divide into about 10,000 elongated sporozoites. This does not occur unless ambient temperatures range from 16 to 33°C. The sporozoites burst out of the oocyst into the haemocoele of the mosquito and the majority migrates to the salivary glands (Gilles and Warrel 1993).

1.1.2.2 Mosquito cycle Anopheles mosquitoes need stagnant water to complete their life cycle comprised of four stages: egg, larva, pupa and adult (Figure 1.3). Only the female mosquito bites since she needs a blood meal to develop her eggs. Each female can develop several hundred eggs at each blood meal and lay them in or around water. The eggs are either attached to each other to form a raft or individually floating on the water. Eggs hatch within 24–48 hours releasing larvae which will change to pupae before becoming adult mosquitoes. The process from eggs to adult mosquito may take one to several weeks depending on the species and the ambient temperature (Jepson et al. 1947, Service 1973). The newly emerged mosquito has to stand on still water to dry its wings before flying away. The female mosquito begins to seek out a human or an animal to feed on several days after emerging from the water. Adult mosquitoes can live for four to eight weeks.

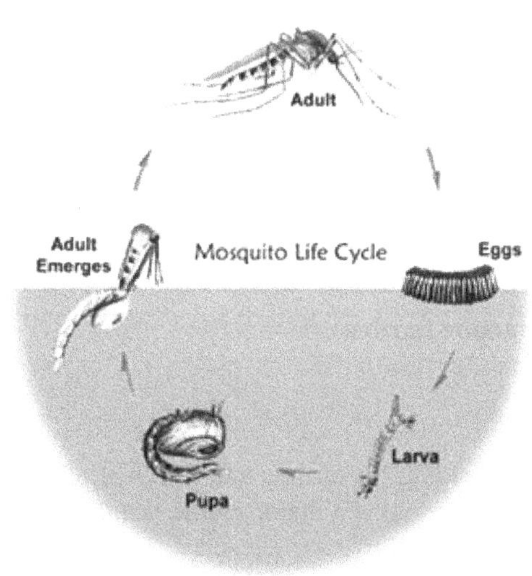

Figure 1.3 Mosquito development cycle

1.1.3 Clinical symptoms

After a bite by an infectious vector, it takes 7 to 30 days before the first symptoms appear. The duration of this period (incubation) depends on the parasite. It is much shorter for *P. falciparum* and longer for *P. malariae*. The first symptoms can be delayed by prophylaxis. The symptoms of malaria vary depending on whether the case is uncomplicated or severe.

In case of uncomplicated malaria, the classical attack lasts from 6 to 10 hours with a cold stage (sensation of cold, shivering). This stage is followed by a hot stage (fever, headaches, vomiting; seizures in young children) and a sweating stage (sweats, return to normal temperature, tiredness). Most often the attacks occur every second day with *P. falciparum*, *P. vivax*, and *P. ovale* and every third day with *P. malariae*. The most common symptoms are a combination of fever chills, sweats, headaches, nausea and vomiting, body aches and general malaise. In endemic areas, physical signs may include perspiration, weakness and enlarged spleen. With *P. falciparum* malaria mild jaundice, enlargement of the liver and increase respiratory rate can be observed.

P. falciparum causes severe malaria and this occurs mainly in individuals with no or low immunity. This includes individuals from unstable and non-malaria areas, children under five years old, pregnant women and tourists. Severe malaria can result in cerebral malaria, with impairment of consciousness, seizures and coma. Other signs are severe anaemia (because of the destruction of red blood cells), pulmonary oedema, and cardiovascular collapse and shock (Taylor 2000).

Although these symptoms give a sensitive diagnosis of malaria, confirmation can only be achieved by laboratory test. Indeed, a definite diagnosis of malaria depends on the presence of parasites on a blood smear examined under microscope or antigen identification through Polymerase Chain Reaction (PCR). In endemic areas the parasite density is sometimes important to define a clinical case of malaria, as low parasitemea in the bloodstream may not cause disease. In an area of high endemicity such as Burkina Faso, a 5,000 parasites per µl plus clinical symptoms is needed to declare clinical malaria (Müller et al. 2001).

1.2 Malaria epidemiology and economic burden

1.2.1 Malaria epidemiology

Despite major achievements in understanding the disease and the great efforts in implementing control strategies, malaria remains a major public health problem worldwide and in Africa (Figure 1.4).

About 41% of the world population is living in malaria endemic regions. The number of clinical cases observed yearly is about 300–500 million (WHO 2002). Out of this number an estimated 1.5–3 million of deaths are observed (Bremen 2001). Sub-Saharan Africa contributes about 90% of deaths, mainly occurring among young children and pregnant women (WHO/UNICEF 2003, Steketee et al. 2001, Bryce et al. 2005).

For decades, several initiatives have been undertaken to control and reduce the malaria burden. Unfortunately, the success of these actions remains restricted to

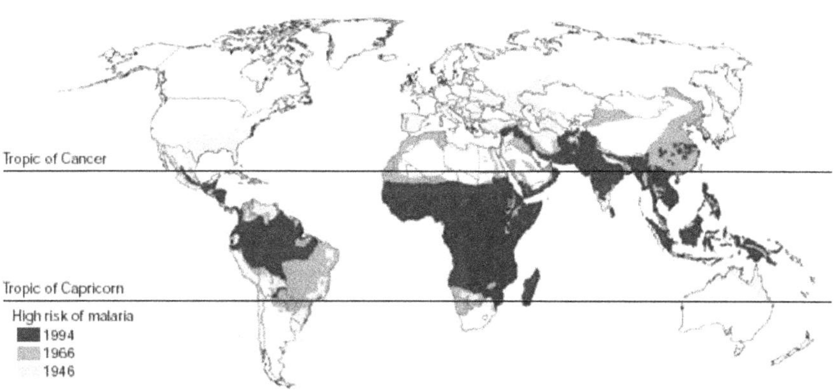

Figure 1.4 Global distribution of malaria (Sachs and Malaney 2002)

some specific areas (WHO 1999). The increase of malaria burden is attributable to several factors. These are parasite resistance to drugs and the mosquito resistance to insecticides (Müller and Garenne 1999, Trapé 2001), breakdown of health care systems, change in agriculture practices, deforestation, and climate changes (Zhou et al. 2005). Without any effective intervention, malaria cases are likely to double over the next 20 years in the high transmission regions (Bremen 2001). Malaria has reappeared in Azerbaijan, Tajikistan, Iraq, and Turkey, where it had previously been under control (Trigg and Kondrachine, 1998a). Regions of Africa situated at a high altitude (>1500 m) were free of malaria until the recent past (Malakooti et al. 1998, Lindblade et al. 2000, Zhou et al. 2005). Since the 1980s, malaria has been increasing (Hay et al. 2002). The reason for this change is a source of controversy. Some argue that climate change is a key determinant (Zhou et al. 2005) whereby a change in climate has led to the increase of temperature in the highlands, and resulted in a suitable environment for mosquito breeding and development. Others think the principal cause is antimalaria drug resistance (Hay et al. 2002) which has undermined control efforts.

Extreme climate events like the El Niño rains of 1997 are followed by malaria outbreaks in semi-arid zones previously free of malaria (WHO 1999). In some regions re-emergence of malaria and epidemics are associated with civil wars, massive population movements and changes in agriculture practice (WHO 1997). Civil war results in the breakdown of the health systems and a concentration of the population in refugee camps. The changes in agriculture practice, like setting up irrigation schemes with standing water creates breeding sites that increase vector population (Sharma & Sharma 1989, Marimbu et al. 1993).

In Burkina Faso, malaria is seasonal, although the transmission is perennial. The highest transmission period coincides with the rainy season (June to December). The overall point prevalence was estimated at 35% among children under five years old (U5s) children (Ministère de la Santé 2001). Malaria represents 20%

of hospital admissions with a case fatality rate of 18% among U5s. In a study in Nouna Health District (north-western Burkina Faso) Müller et al. (2001) reported an incidence of 1.7 episodes per child (age: 6–31 months) during a six-month follow up period. Another study by the same authors found a similar incidence rate of 1.3 (Müller et al. 2003).

1.2.2 Economic and social burden

In tropical regions, malaria affects severely human health and well-being. The daily loss because of malaria is about 2000 children worldwide, making it the third killer among the communicable diseases (Sachs and Malaney 2002). The annual Disability Adjusted Life Years (DALYS), lost because of malaria have been estimated at 35 millions (World Bank 1993). The costs attributable to malaria are high, and countries with high malaria transmission are the poorest in the world. In 1995 the global distribution of per-capita gross domestic product (GDP), after adjusting for Purchasing Power Parity (PPP) showed a correlation between malaria and poverty (Sachs and Malaney 2002). Highly endemic malaria countries have experienced a decline in living standards in the past 30 years and malaria has contributed significantly to this poor economic performance. From 1965 to 1990, the growth rate (0.4%) in per capita GDP/year in these countries was low compared to other developing countries (2.3%) (Gallup and Sachs 2001). Average income GDP (Adjusted for PPP) of high malaria endemic countries was found in 1995 to be five times lower than the one from countries without intensive malaria transmission (US$ 1,526 vs. US$ 8,268) (Gallup and Sachs 2001).

Beyond the economic costs of medical treatment and prevention programmes, there are other costs that directly affect the individual households (Gallup and Sachs 2001). The cost of malaria is substantially high if all related costs were considered. Lost work time, economic losses associated with child sickness and mortality and the cost of treatment and prevention are estimated to be higher than 1% of the countries' gross national product. Further, the economic costs of the pain and suffering associated with the disease are felt to be so high that households might be willing to pay several times the direct income loss caused by malaria to avoid it (Gallup and Sachs 2001).

A household cost of malaria study in Nepal showed that a mean of 6–14 days of work were lost because of malaria (Mills 1993, Over 1993). Since the disease incidence is high during the rainy season when workforce is needed for agriculture work, the loss of productivity is important (Sauerborn et al. 1996). A study estimating the cost of malaria in Rwanda, found that for every US$ 2.28 direct cost per capita because of malaria, 3.6 days of production or 1% of GDP is lost (Ettling and Shepard 1991). In rural Burkina Faso, the total cost was estimated at US$ 0.26 per capita (Sauerborn et al. 1991).

The burden of malaria is high and rising, at the global, regional, national, and individual household level. As a result, the economic losses are estimated as several per cent of GDP in a single year in malaria endemic countries. This raises some questions: Why this high and increasing burden? What are the predictors?

1.3 Risk factors for malaria transmission

Malaria transmission is influenced by several factors that can be grouped into internal and external factors. Internal factors are those characterising the parasite, vector and host susceptibility. They can also be considered as biological factors. External factors include the physical environment, socio-economic and prevention. The different risk factors for malaria have been extensively studied. A review of these studies is given in Table 1.1.

Table 1.1 Summary of malaria risk factors studies

Risk factors	References
Biological: Age Pregnancy Immunity	Steketee et al. 2001, Müller et al. 2001, Lindsay et al. 2000a, Lindsay et al. 2000b, Ansell et al. 2002, Müller et al. 2003, WHO/UNICEF 2003, Okoko et al. 2003, Lusingu et al. 2004, Shanks et al. 2005.
Physical environment: Temperature	Macdonald 1957, Bradley et al. 1987, Detinova 1962, Martens et al. 1995, Lindsay and Birley 1996, Patz et al. 1998, Shililu et al. 1998, Craig et al. 1999, Piebe de vries and Martens 2000, Lindblade et al. 2000, Shanks et al. 2000, Githeko and Ndegwa 2001, Kleinschmidt et al. 2001b, Shanks et al. 2002, Hay et al. 2002, Craig et al. 2004, Teklehaimanot et al. 2004.
Rainfall and humidity	Gill 1920, Haddow 1942, Russell et al. 1963, Pampana 1969, Craig et al. 1999, WHO 1998, Shililu et al. 1998, Lindsay and Martens 1998, Lindblade et al. 1999, Lindsay et al. 2000, Githeko and Ndegwa 2001, Klienschmidt et al. 2001b, Shanks et al. 2002, Teklehaimanot et al. 2004, Zhou et al. 2005.
Land cover	Clements 1999, Patz et al. 1998, Hay et al. 1998, Eisele et al. 2003.
Socioeconomic: Agriculture practices	Sharma and Sharma 1989, Marimbu et al. 1993, Sharma et al. 1994, Singh et al.1996, Lindblade et al. 2000, Baldet et al. 2003, Sissoko et al. 2004, Koudou et al. 2005.
Housing conditions	Gamage-Mendis et al. 1991, Luckner et al. 1998, Snow et al. 1998, Mbogo et al. 1993, Ghebreyesus et al. 2000, Lindsay et al. 2002, Konradsen et al. 2003, Lindsay et al. 2003, Palsson et al. 2004, Okech et al. 2004.
Preventive measures: Insecticide spray, Insecticide treated nets, Repellents, Antimalaria drug	Snow et al. 1997, Doke et al. 2000, Charlwood et al. 2001, Takken 2002, Hawley et al. 2003, Lengeler 2004, Ansari et al. 2004, Cot et al. 2002, Gunasekaran et al. 2005.

1.3.1 Biological factors

Susceptibility to malaria infection depends on individual biological characteristics. In malaria endemic regions, age is an important factor for malaria risk. Younger children are more prone to malaria than adults. Several studies have found a positive correlation between increasing age and a decrease in clinical malaria (Lusingu et al. 2004, Reyburn et al. 2005). This is largely explained by lack of immunity in the young age. The high incidence and case fatality due to malaria in endemic areas are mainly observed among children under five years (WHO/UNICEF 2003, Steketee et al. 2001, Shanks et al. 2005). After this age, acquired partial immunity provides relative protection from severe malaria. However, individuals remain carriers of *P. falciparum.* Therefore defining malaria in endemic areas takes the parasite load into consideration. In their study in Burkina Faso, Müller et al. (2001, 2003) used the threshold of 5,000 parasites per μl. Individuals coming from non-malaria transmission and unstable malaria regions are equally at high-risk independent of their ages. They lack immunity against the parasite and are more likely to experience high case fatality as do children in endemic regions.

Pregnant women are also among the high-risk group. Because of the increased heat and release of volatile substances from their skin surface, they are more attractive to mosquitoes (Lindsay et al. 2000a), therefore increasing their risk of contracting malaria. A study in Eastern Sudan, Himeidan et al. (2004) found that pregnant woman attracted significantly more *Anopheles arabiensis* than non-pregnant women, with higher mean bites per night (0.94 vs. 0.49, $P = 0.005$). Ansell et al. (2002) also found similar results. In addition, pregnancy alters the immune response system, especially for primigravidae women (Okoko et al. 2003).

1.3.2 Socioeconomic factors

1.3.2.1 Housing conditions Several studies have reported housing conditions as an important parameter affecting the incidence *P. falciparum* infection (Gamage-Mendis et al. 1991, Ghebreyesus et al. 2000, Lindsay et al. 2002, Konradsen et al. 2003, Luckner et al. 1998, Snow et al. 1998c). Better constructed houses may act as a natural barrier preventing mosquitoes entering the house. In Sri Lanka, Gamage-Mendis and colleagues showed that, living in a completed house with brick, plaster walls and tiled roofs reduced malaria risk compared to living in a poorly built house (Gamage-Mendis et al. 1991). In rural Gambia, Lindsay et al. (2003) showed that adding ceilings in mud huts reduced the number of Anopheles mosquitoes entering the room and may be an effective way to reduce malaria risk. In Guinea Bissau, Palsson et al. (2004) found a significantly number of Anopheles mosquitoes in houses with open eaves and well in the compound. The presence of animals was also a risk factor for the increase of mosquito abundance (Palsson et al. 2004). The number of people living in a house was associated with increased malaria incidence as well (Mbogo et al. 1993). In Kenya, Okech et al. (2004)

found that indoor temperature variation did not delay the development of malaria parasites in *An. gambiae* and therefore did not impact on malaria transmission.

The location of the house plays as well an important role in malaria transmission. Occupants of houses near an open body of water – a potential breeding site for mosquitoes, are more likely to get malaria than those located faraway (Trapé et al. 1992, Ghebreyesus et al. 1999). Other studies have reported a higher vector density in houses close to breeding sites (Lindsay et al. 1995, Minakawa et al. 2002).

1.3.2.2 Agriculture practices Agriculture is the main sources of income in most of the malaria endemic countries. However, it leads to an important transformation of the ecological landscape, sometimes creating suitable habitats for malaria vectors. In India, introducing intensive irrigation agriculture during the green revolution increased malaria transmission. Some parts of the country changed from epidemic to endemic malaria regions (Sharma and Sharma 1989). Similarly, in Mali and Burkina Faso a higher malaria incidence throughout the year was reported in villages with irrigated rice compared to those without. Because of irrigation, seasonal transmission has now become perennial (Baldet et al. 2003, Sissoko et al. 2004). Another study in India, documented increased malaria transmission in the Thar Desert where until 1980 there were no malaria epidemics despite the significant rains. This increase was attributed to mismanagement of the widespread developmental activities of canal-based irrigation (Singh et al. 1996).

Agricultural practices can also create large areas for stagnant water suitable for mosquito breeding. Rice fields are the best example. A study in rural Central Cote d'Ivoire found a significant decrease of malaria transmission after interrupting irrigated rice growing. Comparing two villages, Koudou et al. (2005) observed that in the village with irrigated rice growing, transmission remains high from February 2002 to August 2003, while in the other one there is a significant decrease in this period. In Burundi, malaria epidemics were associated with local rice fields and fish ponds (Marimbu et al. 1993). However, there are conflicting opinions about whether increases in rice cultivation area correlate with increases in malaria. In the Uganda highlands, Lindblade et al. 2000 did not find significant differences in malaria incidence between the natural swamps and the cultivated (rice) ones. However, the maximum and minimum temperatures were higher in the area near the cultivated swamps. Sharma et al. (1994) did not find a correlation between an increase in rice cultivation area and an increase in malaria transmission. Further studies are needed to better understand the relationship between these two factors.

1.3.2.3 Preventive measures Malaria infection risk can be substantially reduced by proper interventions, whether by reducing the human-vector contact or by giving effective preventive medicine. Insecticide spraying has been shown to reduce significantly the number of mosquitoes and therefore decrease malaria infection (Doke et al. 2000, Ansari and Razdan 2004, Gunasekaran et al.

2005). Dichlorodiphenyl Trichloroethane (DDT) indoor residual spraying in an intervention trial in India was associated with a significant decrease of incidence of malaria fever as well as prevalence of malaria infection (Gunasekaran et al. 2005). However, there are some conflicting views on the effective reduction of malaria infection by insecticide spraying. An intervention trial on the efficacy of indoor spraying on morbidity and mortality in refugee camps in eastern Sudan showed a significant reduction of mortality rates three months after the spray. There was no significant difference in clinical malaria incidence between sprayed and non-sprayed camps (Charlwood et al. 2001).

Insecticide-impregnated mosquito-nets (ITN) have been shown to be effective in reducing human-vector contact and therefore reducing malaria morbidity and mortality among children in malaria endemic areas (Hawley et al. 2003, Lengeler 2004). However there are some concerns about the long-term effects. In high endemic areas, ITN may interfere with the development of partial immunity leading to higher susceptibility to severe malaria (Snow et al. 1997, Modiano et al. 1998). Questions have also been raised about the risk of vectors changing their feeding behaviour, to earlier biting when the host is accessible, in the presence of ITN (Takken 2002).

Preventive medicine reduces the risk of severe malaria by keeping the parasite density in humans low. It is recommended in endemic areas for high-risk groups, such as children below five years and pregnant women. For maximum efficacy in reducing malaria incidence, all preventions should be combined (Cot et al. 2002).

1.3.3 Physical environment

1.3.3.1 Temperature Ambient temperature plays a major role in the malaria vector life cycle. The development of the parasite within the mosquito (sporogonic cycle) depends on temperature. The time delay between infection of the mosquito and the infectious stage is estimated at 9–10 days at temperatures of 28°C, while development stops at temperatures below 16°C (Macdonald 1957, Bradley et al. 1987). Figure 1.5a shows the rapid decrease of the sporogonic cycle length with increase in temperature. At 28°C the cycle length is shorter (Lindsay and Birley 1996). Daily vector survival (90%) is stable at temperatures between 16 and 36°C. Higher temperature increases mosquito mortality (Figure 1.5b). The number of mosquitoes surviving the sporogonic cycle shows a bell-shaped relationship with temperature (Figure 1.5c). At low temperatures the vector needs to survive long enough for the sporogonic cycle to take place and at high temperature the mosquitoes survive less. The highest proportion of vectors surviving the incubation period is observed at temperature between 28° and 32°C (Craig et al. 1999). The gonotrophic cycle, which is the vector feeding interval, is shortened by high temperature (Figure 1.5d). Since high temperatures increase the digestion rate of blood meals, this results in more frequent vector-host contacts.

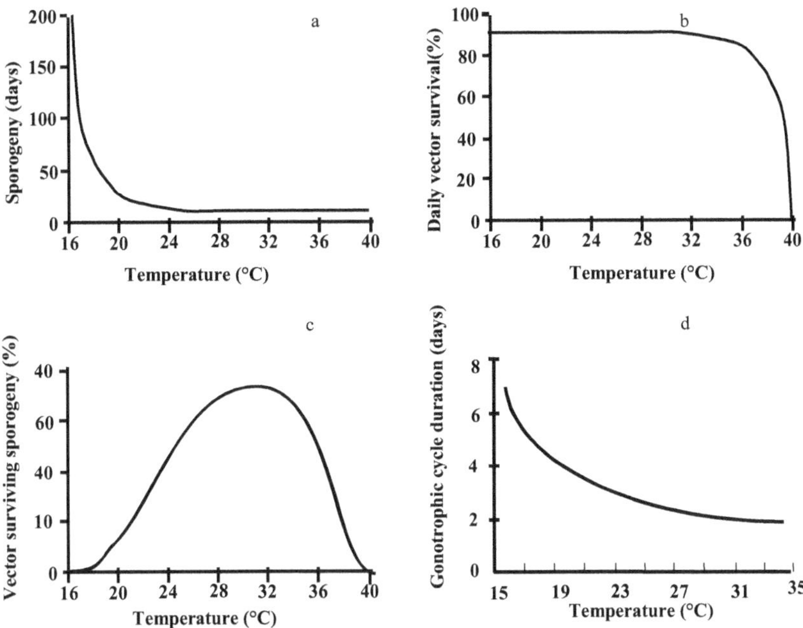

Figure 1.5 **Effect of ambient temperature on malaria vector adult stage: (a) duration of the sporogonic cycle in days (Macdonald 1957, Detinova, 1962); (b) daily mosquito survival (Martens 1997); (c) percentage of vectors surviving sporogeny; (d) gonotrophic cycle (Detinova, 1962)**

Immature stages of the vector are equally temperature dependent (Figure 1.6a and 1.6b). The duration of the larval stage is long at 16°C and consistently decreases with the increase of temperature. The shortest time is observed at 36 °C (Figure 1.6b). This relationship is expressed by Detinova as:

$$n = \frac{111}{T°C - 18},$$

where n is the duration in days of the larval stage, T°C the ambient temperature, 18°C the threshold below which larval development stops and 111 is the thermal sum in degree-days (Detinova 1962).

Temperature is therefore the main determinant of the basic reproduction rate (R_0) which is defined as the expected new infections per case without immunity. Mathematically, R_0 is expressed as:

$$R_0 = \frac{ma^2bp^n}{-r(\log_e p)}$$

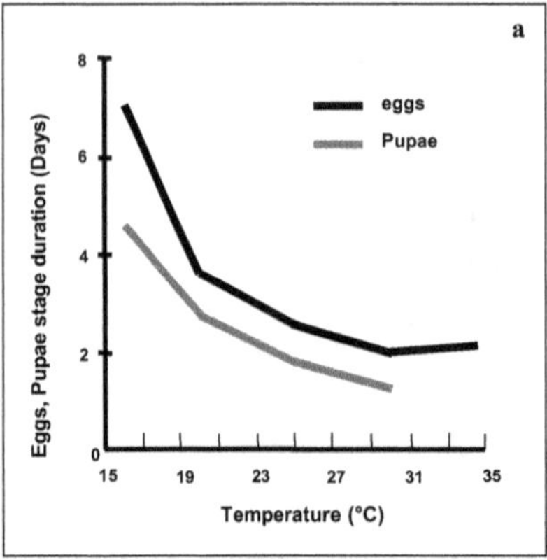

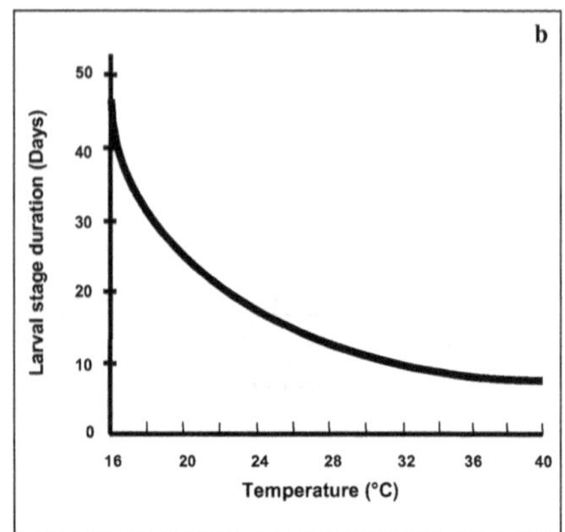

Figure 1.6 Ambient temperature and malaria vector immature stage: eggs Pupae (a), larvae (b) from Jepson et al. 1947 and le Sueur et al. 1997

where *ma* is the human biting rate, *b* the proportion of vector females developing parasites, *p* the probability of vector survival through the sporogonic period and *r* the rate of recovery of humans from infection. If $R_0 < 1$, malaria will die out; if $R_0 > 1$ malaria will spread indefinitely (Macdonald 1957). Malaria Transmission Potential (TP), derived from the (R_0) uses temperature as an important parameter. This formula is defined as:

$$TP = \frac{bca^2p^n}{-\ln(p)};$$

where *n* is the incubation period of the parasite in the malaria infected mosquito and determined by minimum and maximal temperature (Martens et al. 1995). The parasite develops in the mosquito within a specific temperature range. The minimum temperature for *P. falciparum* ranges between 10 and 16°C. An increase in the temperature increases the potential of rapid development of the parasite, but at temperatures over 32–34°C the survival rate decreases (Piebe de vries and Martens 2000).

Several field studies have shown the impact of ambient temperature on malaria outcomes. (Patz et al. 1998, Shililu et al. 1998, Lindblade et al. 2000, Githeko and Ndegwa 2001, Shanks et al. 2002, Craig et al. 2004, Teklehaimanot et al. 2004, Zhou et al. 2005). Craig et al. (2004), compared clinical malaria data over 30 years with climate in KwaZulu-Natal (KZN), South Africa and found significant correlation of temperature and malaria cases. Mean maximum daily temperatures from January to October of the preceding season were positively associated with clinical cases of malaria ($r^2 = 0.364$). Another study in Ethiopia compared ten years of microscopically confirmed *P. falciparum* cases from health facilities to meteorological data from local stations. The authors found that minimum temperature was associated with malaria in a cold district (minimum temperature below 12°C), while in the hot ones (minimum temperature above 12°C) the effect was not significant (Teklehaimanot et al. 2004).

Because of the impact of temperature on malaria, global warming may lead to increased risk of malaria among the world population. However, this opinion is controversial. In Kenya, Shanks et al. (2000) could not find a link between ambient temperature and malaria admissions over a 30-year period, as there were no significant trends in average monthly temperature or mean monthly rainfall over the period of study. Similarly, Hay et al. (2002) explained the increase of malaria morbidity in four sites of East Africa as being because of drug resistance, rather than changes in temperature. Patz (2002) argues that this discrepancy may rise from methodological issues. In these studies, climate data were derived from interpolating a broad-scale gridded regional climate dataset based on sparse historical weather station data which is unsuitable for individual village sites (Patz 2002). Kovats et al. (2001) described this as an "absence of evidence, rather than evidence of absence of a (climate) effect." For assessing climate and infectious disease outcomes they recommended: "(i) evidence for biological sensitivity to climate, requiring both field and laboratory research on important vectors and pathogens; (ii) meteorological evidence of climate change, requiring sufficient measurements for specific study regions; and (iii) evidence for epidemiological or entomological change with climate change, accounting for potential confounding factors" (Kovats et al. 2001).

1.3.3.2 Rainfall and humidity Most malaria vectors depend on rainfall, since it provides breeding sites for the mosquitoes to lay their eggs. Rainfall also ensures suitable relative humidity of at least 50–60% for mosquitoes' survival. A relative humidity value below 60% shortens the life-span of the mosquitoes. However, too much rain in the form of storms can destroy breeding sites or flush away the eggs or larvae (Pampana 1969, Craig et al. 1999).

In the early days of malaria research, rainfall was already associated with malaria. The onset of the rainy season was correlated with an increase in vector abundance (Gill 1920, Haddow 1942). From 1921, the forecasts for malaria epidemics in north-east of Pakistan and north-west India were based on the proved relationship between rainfall and malaria mortality (WHO 1998). The 1958 malaria epidemic outbreak in Ethiopia was associated with unusually high amounts of rain. Similarly in Nairobi, Kenya outbreaks of malaria occurred in 1940 after heavy rains (Lindsay and Martens 1998). In the Ugandan highlands, rainfall anomalies (difference from the mean) because of the 1997 El Niño were positively correlated with vector density one month later and this may have initiated the resulting epidemic (Lindblade et al. 1999). The association between rainfall and malaria was consistently observed in several others studies (Githeko and Ndegwa 2001, Teklehaimanot et al. 2004, Zhou et al. 2005). Nonetheless, in some studies the rainfall-malaria relationship was not established. Lindsay et al. (2000b) found in Tanzania highlands that after one El Niño event with 2.4 times more rainfall than normal, there was less malaria than the year before.

Malaria vector survival is also affected by the distribution of rainfall throughout the year, whether in the wet or dry season. During the wet season, rainwater remains on the surface and provides a place for mosquitoes to breed and a chance for the larvae to complete their development cycle. In contrast, rainwater during the dry season evaporates rapidly and does not stay long enough to provide mosquito larva habitats (Russell et al. 1963).

Despite this, rainfall is not always associated with malaria transmission risk (Shililu et al. 1998, Shanks et al. 2002). Some vectors such as *An. funestus* prefer to breed in permanent habitats (Gillies and Coetzee 1987). Furthermore, the increase of vector density, because of rainfall, may induce the population to protect itself from mosquito nuisance, therefore reducing malaria incidence.

1.3.3.3 Land cover Land cover, in particular vegetation has been associated with malaria transmission, because it provides suitable environment for mosquito breeding. The presence of vegetation creates microclimatic conditions (moderate temperature and humidity) suitable for mosquitoes (Clements 1999). Land cover can be measured directly by field observation or indirectly by satellite imagery. Satellite imagery can quantify the amount of vegetation by the Normative Difference Vegetation Index (NDVI). It is derived from the Spectral Vegetation Indices (SVI) which exploits the light reflectance of the vegetation.
Land-Sat Thematic Mapper (TM), NDVI is expressed as:

$$NDVI = \frac{Channel4 - Channel2}{Channel4 + Channel2}.$$

The result is a ratio with a value between -1 and +1, but in practice values are recorded within the limits, 0.0–0.2.

In Kenya, NDVI was found to be correlated with human biting rate (Patz et al. 1998), and with annual malaria cases (Hay et al. 1998). At spatial resolution of 270 metres × 270 metres, Eisele et al. (2003) successfully described the variations in entomological and human ecological parameters. Given the household density, the number of potential Anopheles larval habitats increased with increasing mean value of NDVI.

NDVI is a good proxy for assessing the effect of land cover on malaria transmission; although note that field validation is required for better estimates.

1.3.3.4 Assessing malaria risk Measuring malaria risk has been a concern since the discovery of the link between mosquito and the parasite. Macdonald (1957) introduced the "basic reproductive rate" concept to describe the sustainability of malaria transmission. As already described (section 1.3.3.1), it expresses the number of new infections from a single case of malaria without immunity. Malaria transmission is sustained if this number is above one (Macdonald 1957). This concept includes the parasitological and mosquitoes aspect. Vectorial Capacity (VC) was later introduced by Garrett-Jones (1964), who removed the parasitological aspect from the "basic reproductive rate". The VC expresses the daily expected inoculation of humans per infective case. The most commonly used concept to measure malaria transmission under field conditions is the Entomological Inoculation Rate (EIR). It is defined as the number of infective bites per person per night (Onori and Grab 1980). In Eritrea, Shililu et al. (2003) used EIR to show that the risk of exposure to infected mosquitoes was heterogeneous and seasonal, with high inoculation rates during rainy-season, and with little or no transmission during the dry season. They concluded that EIR can help in quantifying levels of exposure in different regions of the country and could be used for evaluating the vector control programmes (Shililu et al. 2003). Although, the relationship between EIR and malaria outcome risk had been demonstrated in several studies (Beier et al. 1994, Beier et al. 1999, Smith et al. 2001), there are still some controversies. In endemic areas high EIR may not necessary lead to high malaria morbidity or mortality as exposed population may develop immunity and thus be less susceptible to malaria attacks.

Malaria risk can also be measured by parasite prevalence (number of infected hosts) or by parasite incidence (number of newly infected hosts). Since parasite prevalence in endemic area is not always an expression of clinical malaria, morbidity (number of clinically sick persons) can be used a measure of malaria risk. These different measures can be used to compare different geographical settings, different periods (rainy and dry season, before and after intervention). Table 1.2 gives an overview of malaria risk assessment methods.

Table 1.2 Malaria risk parameters (Gilles and Warrel 1993)

Parameters	Definition of index	Methods	Formula
Human biting Rate (HBR)	Bites per person per night by vector population	Human bait capture. *a*, mosquito feeding frequency *m*, human blood index HBI	ma
Vectorial capacity (VC)	Expected inoculations of human per infective case per time unit	*ma* (HBR), *p* daily mosquito population survival *n*, incubation period of parasite in vector	$\frac{ma^2p^n}{-\ln p}$
Basis reproductive rate (R_0)	Expected new infections per cases without immunity	*b*, % of vector developing parasite following ingestion of gametes *r* recovery rate from infection	$\frac{ma^2bp^n}{-r\ln p}$
Entomological Inoculation rate (EIR)	Number of infective bites per person per time unit	*ma* (HBR), *s* proportion of infected mosquitoes (sporozoite rate)	mas
Parasite prevalence	% of infected person	Laboratory test	
Morbidity (Prevalence/ Incidence)	% of clinical malaria cases or number of new cases during a given period	Laboratory test and clinical examination	

1.4 Fighting malaria

1.4.1 Control strategies

Several control measures have been implemented including prevention and treatment. The most important was the malaria eradication programme implemented after the Second World War with the discovery of Dichlorodiphenyl Trichloroethane, (DDT), an effective insecticide product (Najera 1989, Onori et al. 1993, Müller 2000). This programme was decided after the eighth World Health Assembly in 1945. It comprised large-scale application of DDT, the use of the insecticide to reduce mosquito population and treating presumptive cases of malaria. The programme was successful in eradicating malaria in some regions such as Europe, Asia, the former USSR, the Middle East, North and South America and the Caribbean. However, it was less successful in Africa and some Asians countries (Trigg and Kondrachine 1998b). The failure was attributed to the lack of infrastructure (road and health), restricting the programme to Ethiopia, South Africa, Zimbabwe, then Southern Rhodesia (Najera 1989, Müller 2000), the development of insecticide resistance by the mosquito and the development of resistance by the parasites to antimalaria drugs (Lepes 1974).

In 1969, the World Health Assembly reaffirmed the malaria eradication goals with a new strategy focusing on the regions where eradication was not achieved. This strategy, based on national control programmes has suffered from lack of resources, because of the perceived failure of the eradication programme that led to decrease of external funding. This situation was aggravated by the economic crisis in the 1970s which led to a dramatic increase in the costs of drugs and insecticides. The result of this situation is the resurgence of malaria in many regions of south Asia and Latin America (Müller 2000).

The global status of malaria programmes, in 1979 showed that, eradication was effective only in 37 countries out of 143 countries previously endemic. The risk was reduced in 16 countries and the disease remained a major public health problem in 90 countries. Because of this the 31st World Health Organization conference recommended strategies for malaria control following the principle of Primary Health Care (PHC) introduced a year previously at the Alma-Ata conference. The idea was developing PHC which would ensure the basic health for malaria control. Unfortunately, this approach also had limits (Najera 1989) and the malaria problem increased during the 1980s (WHO 1997).

In 1992, WHO implemented a new approach, based on a comprehensive global strategy integrating PHC, decentralisation and multisectoral approaches (WHO 1993). The technical elements (four pillars of malaria control), of this strategy are:

- to provide early diagnosis and prompt treatment;
- to plan and implement selective and sustainable preventive measures, including vector control;

- to detect, contain, or prevent epidemics;
- to strengthen local capacities in basic and applied research;
- τo allow and promote the regular assessment of country's malaria situation in particular the ecological social and economic determinants of the disease.

The Roll Back Malaria Initiative (RBM) was launched in 1998 in Abuja-Nigeria to strengthen these strategies. The main aim was to reduce by half mortality due to malaria by 2010, in line with the Millennium Development Goals (MDG) by developing a new, sector-wide partnership to combat the disease at global, regional, country and local levels.

Malaria control strategies have undergone changes over time to respond to the increases of the disease burden. Unfortunately, no strategies have been able to stop the increasing spread of malaria. Eradication of the disease in the short-term is a dream, but proper and comprehensive strategies for control programmes need to be designed and implemented. The increasing interest in developing prediction, forecasting and early warning tools will be helpful. The question remains on how to integrate these new technologies in a comprehensive strategy.

1.4.2 Modelling malaria transmission

Malaria transmission modelling involves non-spatial and spatial components. The non-spatial models address the basic epidemiological questions: Will malaria cause an epidemic? Can malaria persist in a population? When will malaria epidemics occur and reoccur? The spatial-models predict where malaria transmission is likely to occur based on environmental factors.

1.4.2.1 Non-spatial modelling In 1760, Bernoulli introduced mathematical modelling in the study of infectious diseases (Dietz and Heesterbeek 2002). He used mathematical methods to evaluate the effectiveness of the technique of variolation against smallpox (Anderson and May 1991). Further applications have been done with this approach, but modern mathematical epidemiology owes much to the work of Ross, Soper, Kermack and McKendrick. They began to develop specific theories about the transmission of infectious diseases in precise mathematical statements and to investigate the proprieties of the resulting models (Ross 1911, Kermack and McKendrick 1927, Soper 1929). Their work led to one of the cornerstones of modern mathematical epidemiology with the hypothesis that the course of an epidemic depends on the rate of contact between susceptible and infectious individuals.

The first mathematical model for malaria transmission was developed by Ronald Ross to predict the spread of the diseases (Ross 1911). Ross later concluded that to eradicate malaria, we do not need to eliminate the mosquito vector, but to increase its mortality (Ross 1928). Further, he insisted that successful control programmes should not only be based on one aspect, but should rather integrate vector decrease (larvicides), drug treatment (quinine), and personal protection (mosquito nets) (Ross 1928). Unfortunately, Ross' conclusions got little attention from his contemporaries (Utzinger et al. 2001). In the 1950s, George Macdonald, building on Ross' models, concluded that at equilibrium, the weakest link in malaria transmission cycle was the survival of adult female Anopheles (Macdonald 1957). The conclusion led to the global malaria eradication campaign based on DDT spraying, with DDT targeted at adult female Anopheles. Macdonald's model was based on the basic assumption that vector and human hosts could be subdivided into susceptible, infected and infectious (Figure 1.7).

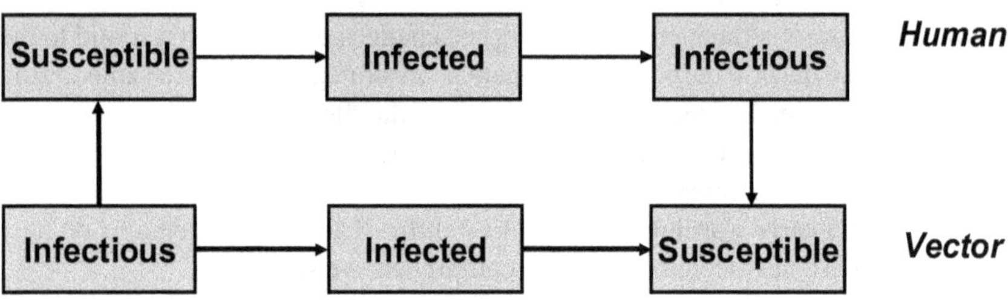

Figure 1.7 Schematic representation of the Ross-Macdonald model

In the 1970s, Dietz and Molineaux (1974) further improved the simple Macdonald model by clearly considering human immunity interacting with the transmission dynamics (Molineaux and Gramiccia 1980). In the Garki project, they developed a more sophisticated model (Garki model). According to them, this model was "realistic" in its ability to simulate malaria epidemiology at Garki, given entomologic inputs, and it provided comparative forecasts for several specific interventions (McKenzie and Samba 2004). The Garki model included age-specific prediction of malaria prevalence as a function of the vectorial capacity (VC), defined as the number of potentially infective contacts induced by the mosquito population per infectious person per day. (Dietz et al. 1974) The model described transitions of the host in seven stages characterised by infection and immunological status (Figure 1.8).

Further, Halloran and colleagues explicitly considered the population-level effects of potential stage-specific vaccines (Halloran et al. 1989). From there malaria modelling has gained attention. The development of computers allowed the basic ideas of the compartment models to be taken down to individual level. Populations are modelled as large numbers of interacting individual humans and individual mosquitoes, each with its own characteristics and dynamics (Mckenzie and Samba 2004). Further steps toward biological realism have begun to include the effects of weather (Hoshen and Morse 2005), meiotic recombination

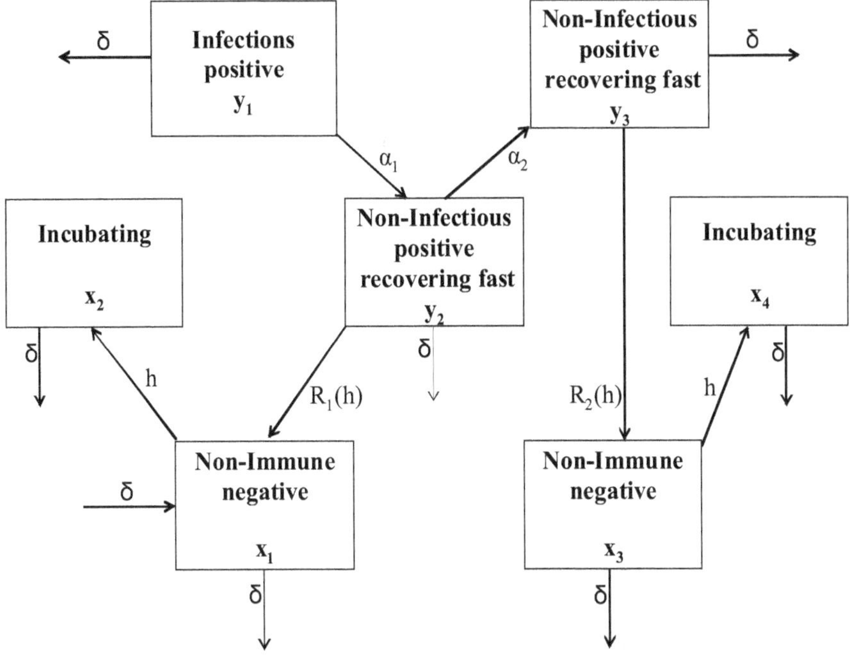

Figure 1.8 States and transitions in the Garki model

Note: x_1 and x_3, are the uninfected individuals, and x_2 and x_4 are the infected individuals, $y_{1,}$ y_2 and y_3, represent proportions of humans with blood-stage infections. The model predicts the proportion of the human population at each age in each of the compartments. It is defined by a set of linked difference equations (Annex 1) that define the changes in each of these proportions.

among parasites, immunologic cross-reactivity, and other factors (McKenzie et al. 2002).

Many contemporary malaria models focus on the connection between weather, which determines vector survival and abundance, and malaria prevalence. Such models are typically statistical (Randolph and Rogers 2000, Kleinschmidt et al. 2001a, Hay et al. 2002, Rogers et al. 2002), Fuzzy logic (Craig et al. 1999, MARA/ARMA 1998), rule based (Martens et al. 1995, Lindsay and Martens 1998) or process based (Macdonald 1965, Dietz 1988, Lindsay and Birley 1996). While the first three methods are well-developed, they do not have the ability to predict the impact of changing conditions (environmental or resistance pattern) or human intervention (McKenzie 2000).

Non-spatial modelling of malaria is appropriate for prediction in point and time, but less suitable for its spatial distribution. It however supports spatial modelling which can extrapolate from point prediction.

1.4.2.2 Spatial modelling of malaria Spatial modelling of malaria transmission is an important tool to support control strategies. It helps to identify high-risk geographical areas and the most important predictor for malaria transmission among the environmental variables. Further, spatial modelling can be used to better understand the interaction between environmental factors and their impact on malaria risk. Spatial modelling uses Geographical Information Systems (GIS), Remote Sensing (RS) tools and statistical methods to produce risk maps.

1.4.3 Geographical Information Systems and Remote Sensing

1.4.3.1 Geographical Information Systems and malaria Geographical information systems are computer hardware and software packages which are used for capturing, storing, manipulating, querying, displaying and analysing all types of geographical information (DeMers 1997, Burrough and McDonnell 1998). A typical GIS database contains descriptive information about spatial features and the internal and external topological connections. GIS are characterised by the strict link between a feature's geographical position (co-ordinate) and its attribute data. This allows users to manipulate, analyse and query information on various map features through their shared components. The power of GIS is its ability to integrate and manipulate multiple layers or themes of spatial data for a large area and from different sources at different scales. GIS data sources are paper maps, aerial photographs, satellite images, Geographical Positioning Systems (GPS) as well as routine data, censuses, epidemiological surveys, environmental data, health data and any other data with spatial component. The data have to be registered geographically to a coded common frame of reference (usually a geodetic co-ordinate system) before they can be stored in a GIS. By making easy the manipulation and possible combination of several data layers from the different data sources, GIS allows the rapid display and analysis of multivariate spatial data. GIS is a potentially powerful tool for epidemiology, in mapping diseases and their determinants, quantifying risk, linking diseases and their potential risk factors, and creating databases for further statistical and epidemiological analyses.

In health, GIS is able to help us understand how health problems are spatially distributed and related environmental factors (Loslier 1995). For malaria research and control, GIS has great potential since it has the capacity to integrate information on all aspects of malaria including the environmental factors, infrastructure and demography. It provides a stratification of the disease for targeted intervention programmes (Brêtas 1995, Carter et al. 2000). GIS has been intensively used in malaria research to examine the link between environmental factors and malaria transmission risk (Kitron et al. 1994, Omumbo et al. 1998, Schellenberg et al. 1998, Booman et al. 2000, Carter et al. 2000, Rogers et al. 2002, Craig et al.1999, Hay et al. 2002, Van der Hoek et al. 2003, Hassan et al. 2003).

In Israel, Kitron et al. (1994) used GIS to set up a surveillance system for malaria control. Anopheles mosquitoes breeding sites were linked to imported malaria cases to assess the risk of malaria transmission. The GIS-based surveillance system ensured quick identification of localised outbreaks allowing prompt control measures to be most efficiently implemented (Kitron et al. 1994). Using GIS and RS, in India, Sharma and Srivastava showed a correlation between malaria annual parasite incidence and water table, soil type, irrigation and water quality (Sharma and Srivastava 1997). Omumbo et al. (1998) used GIS to quantify the relationship between occurrence of anopheles mosquitoes and environmental variables and Carter et al. (2000) used one to explore the geographical relationship between malaria risk and vector breeding sites. Using GIS, in South Africa, Booman et al. were able to stratify malaria risk in Barbeton and Nkomazi districts. This stratification showed a gradient from West to East within which the risk increased towards the Mozambique border (RR=4.12 95% CI, 3.88–4.46) compared with the remaining areas in these two districts (Booman et al. 2000). Snow et al. (1998a) produced maps of malaria transmission risk of Africa using climate modelling and GIS. Rogers and colleagues were able to predict the EIR of different species of *An gambiae*, using GIS and environmental factors in Africa (Rogers et al. 2002).

In summary, GIS is a powerful tool which can help epidemiologists and public health experts for malaria control to assess the spatial aspects of malaria transmission. Further, it is a good tool of communication to support the decision making (Sauerborn and Karam 2000). Mapping the features of disease in GIS will help malaria researchers to answer the questions: Where is the problem and what spatial patterns exist? What has changed overtime?

1.4.3.2 Remote Sensing and malaria risk prediction Remote sensing is the science and art of obtaining information about an object, area, or phenomenon through the analysis of data acquired by a sensor that is faraway from the units under investigation (Lillesand and Kiefer 1994, Hay et al. 2000). The sensors are mostly cameras, satellite-borne multispectral scanners or radar. The sensors are mounted on a “platform” from a few metres high, or aircrafts, rocket and space shuttle thousands of metres away, or through satellites hundreds or thousands of kilometres above the subjects of interest. Most notable are aircraft, earth-orbiting satellites such as Landsat, the “Satellite Pour l’Observation de la Terre” (SPOT) series, and polar-orbiting meteorological satellites such as National Oceanographic and Atmospheric Administration Advanced Very-High-Resolution Radiometers (NOAA-AVHRR) and Meteosat, High Resolution Radiometer (HRR). The science of remote sensing is based on an object that reflects, absorbs and emits energy at specific and distinctive wavelengths in the electromagnetic spectrum. Passive sensors, including cameras and multispectral scanners, record reflected or emitted energy, while active sensors such as radar send microwave energy to the subject, and then record the returned signal.

The spatial resolution and temporal resolution of the satellite observation varies according to the satellite. Spatial resolution is the size of the smallest object that can be identified; and temporal resolution the time between two observations of the same spot on the surface of the earth. Earth observation satellites can produce a spatial resolution of 1–4 m (Ikonos-2); 10–20 (SPOT); 30–120 m

(Landsat 1–5); 15–60 m (Landsat 7); 250–1000 m (Moderate Resolution Imaging Spectroradiometer (MODIS). Meteorological Satellites have lower spatial resolution with pixel sizes of 1.1 km (NOAA-AVHRR). The temporal resolution of Ikonos is 11 days, 15 for MODIS, 16 for Landsat and 26 for SPOT (Rogers et al. 2002). Remote sensing provides the capability to collect uniform measurements in digital form over large areas at high-speed and to analyse that could not be monitored in any other way (Aronoff 1989). Although remote sensing had been argued to be a useful tool for epidemiological studies of vector-borne diseases for a long-time, the technology in combination with GIS has only been recently extensively used in malaria research.

Sharma and colleagues used the Indian Remote Sensing satellite to study the mosquito distribution around Delhi, India. Water bodies with marshy areas vegetation and human settlement were considered to be responsible for mosquito abundance. Supervised classification was used to produce land use and land cover maps. A survey of larval and adult mosquito density was performed concurrently in the study sites. Results indicated the spatial variation of mosquito densities was positively correlated with water bodies and vegetation in some study sites (Sharma et al. 1996, Sharma and Srivastava 1997).

Hay et al. (1998) used the NDVI, Land Surface Temperature (LST) and Cold Cloud Day (CCD) data derived from NOAA-AVHRR and Meteosat-HRR to model malaria seasonality in community sites in Kenya. They compared the satellite derived variables with the mean percentage of total annual malaria admissions recorded in each month. They found the NDVI in the preceding month correlated most significantly and consistently with malaria presentations across the three sites.

In the Gambia, Thomson et al. (1999) using the Famine Early Warning Systems and spatial statistics, showed a significant association between age related malaria in Gambian children and seasonal environmental greenness (NDVI) derived from satellite data. The model was then used to predict changes in malaria prevalence among children given different mosquito net control scenarios.

Another study in the Gambia used satellite images to examine local-scale variation in malaria transmission and infection in children within a continuous landscape by retrospective spatial analysis of entomological and clinical data collected during 1988 and 1989. Multispectral SPOT satellite imagery at 20-metre spatial resolution was used to map mosquito-breeding habitats retrospectively from 1988. The risk of exposure to the malaria parasite was estimated in 26 villages in rural Gambia based on spatial and clinical data. The results showed that, with increasing exposure, there was an increase of the parasite prevalence, but at higher levels of exposure, parasite prevalence declined. It also showed differences in exposure to malaria in villages over distances of less than 2 km from mosquito breeding sites (Thomas and Lindsay 2000)

Other studies (Randolph and Rogers 2000, Rogers et al. 2002, Nihei et al. 2002, Eisele et al. 2003) have shown the appropriateness of RS techniques for national malaria control programmes.

1.4.3.3 Spatial modelling of malaria risk Mapping spatial and temporal distribution of diseases and their potential determinants is not recent. Historically, mapping diseases has provided important clues to the aetiology of diseases. Snow (1855) developed his hypothesis on the mode of cholera transmission by mapping the association between cholera death and water supply companies in London, as well as the association with London's Broad Street Water pump (Figure 1.9).

Spatial analysis was limited to plotting the observed disease cases or rates and this restricted the analysis to the points where data were available. The development of computers, GIS, RS and statistical methods, allowed an integrated approach with the final aim to extrapolate or predict disease risk for areas where data are not always available. This approach is useful in malaria research, as data are often lacking, and when available, are sparse and localised. The production of malaria maps is therefore based on statistical modelling methods for area-wide prediction of risk. Because of the lack of infection data, malaria risk prediction relies on the proper knowledge of environmental and climatic factors that are driving the transmission (Craig et al. 1999). However, the estimation is complicated by there is often local variation of risk that cannot easily be accounted for by the known covariates. Further, data points of measured malaria prevalence are not evenly

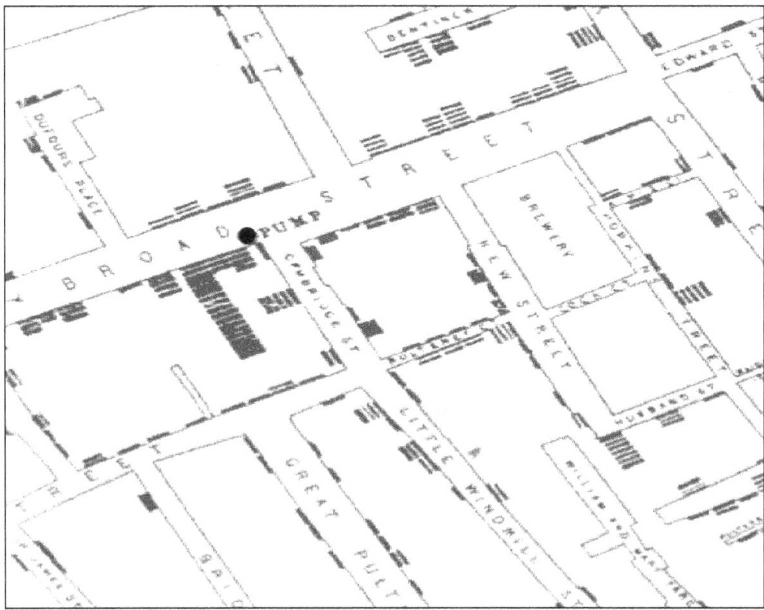

Figure 1.9 John Snow's Cholera map, (Snow 1855) by plotting the deaths (bold line parallel to the building front in which the people died), Dr Snow was able to trace the spread of Cholera to the pump (dot) at the corner of Cambridge and Broad Street

or randomly distributed across a country, or region, but are clustered in areas of high-risk. Any modelling of risk has to consider the spatial autocorrelation of the data, and allow for local deviation from predictions that are based on the known climatic covariates (Kleinschmidt et al. 2000).

Malaria spatial modelling resulting in risk maps is important in supporting control programmes. High-risk areas can be identified and intervention priorities set therefore. Several attempts to predict malaria at different scales have been made (Thomson et al.1997, Snow et al. 1998a, Craig et al. 1999, Kleinschmidt et al. 2000, Thomson et al.1999, Rogers et al. 2002).

Snow et al. (1998a) used a fuzzy logic climate suitability model to define areas of Kenya unsuitable for stable transmission. Using empirical data on *P. falciparum* infection rate among children, they produced a climate-based statistical model of malaria transmission intensity in stable malaria transmission areas. The model was able to identify 75% of three endemicity classes (low, intermediate and high). Applying the model to weather and remote sensing data using GIS, they provided an estimate of the malaria endemicity for all the fourth-level administrative regions in Kenya.

Kleinschmidt et al. (2001b) used the risk-mapping approach to produce an empirical malaria distribution map for West Africa. They used spatial statistical analysis of malaria parasites in relation to environmental factors involved in distributing malaria transmission. This model was then used to predict parasite prevalence in West Africa and to estimate the proportion of each country's population in the region exposed to various categories of health-related problems.

The most comprehensible malaria modelling and prediction in Africa was done by the Mapping Malaria Risk in Africa initiative (MARA/ARMA 1998). GIS was used to model and map the malaria risk in the whole continent of Africa (le Sueur et al. 1997). They used fuzzy logic climate suitability to model the malaria transmission in Africa, based on biological constraints of temperature and rainfall, on malaria parasites and their vector development (Craig et al. 1999). The continental malaria suitability map derived from the fuzzy logic climate suitability model compared well with contemporary field data and historical "expert opinion" maps. They combined a review of the literature on malaria surveys in Africa and the resulting continental risk map derived from the fuzzy logic model to estimate malaria morbidity and mortality in Africa (Omumbo et al. 1998). This was a great achievement and a useful tool for national malaria control programmes. However, the scale (5km*5km) on which the prediction was made is unlikely to provide accurate information about within-country malaria risk differentials, since malaria transmission is dependent on local environmental conditions, which determine the vector dynamics.

In summary, modelling malaria transmission risk is with no doubt an important tool for better control strategies. The development of GIS, RS and mathematical as well as statistical modelling provides a great opportunity to address the spatial and non-spatial aspects of malaria transmission. Though these two components can be modelled separately, the combination produces a more powerful tool for prediction, forecasting and early warning systems.

Although malaria is a global concern and needs global synergy, it is more informative if risks predictions are made at the local scale, as the biological process of transmission dynamics are location dependent. Unfortunately there are few or almost no attempts for local scale prediction. This is because the data needed are not available or enough for good prediction. Interpolations are therefore made based on pooling continental, regional or country data giving less accurate prediction (Kovats et al. 2001). Local scale modelling needs systematic and comprehensive collection of data on all factors involved in malaria transmissions as discussed in section 3.1.

1.5 Rationale of the study

While modelling of malaria transmission risk has been done extensively in East Africa, there are few studies in West Africa. In Burkina Faso where malaria remains endemic, the disease is associated with about 20% of all mortality of children under five years in malaria endemic health districts like Nouna (Nouna Health District 1999). Malaria contribution to the total burden of disease (BOD) in Nouna health district is estimated at 27.7% followed by diarrhoea 20.5% (Wurthwein et al. 2001). Among children under five, it accounts for 1719.5 years of life lost (YLL) out of a total 3033.9 YLL because of malaria for all ages. Since the 1980s, the country has been involved in various studies aimed at identifying locally appropriate methods for controlling the disease. The environmental aspects of malaria transmission remain fully unexplored and little has been done in malaria risk prediction. The seasonal change of the weather, driving the transmission, be, so far, the best way of guessing malaria transmission intensity (Traoré 2003). Few or no attempts have been made to quantify the association between weather and malaria outcomes. Most of the studies have focused mainly on a point estimate of the transmission, without the spatial and time dimensions. Although malaria is endemic in the country, there is significant local variation of transmission intensity. Malaria outcomes driven by local environmental conditions might be informative to capture. Further, malaria control strategies rely on early detection and treatment; therefore prior identification of populations at risk and the periods to intervene will be useful for better allocation of resources for malaria control. In this study we tried to fill this gap by developing a local prediction model (non-spatial and spatial) of malaria risk using village-specific ground-based weather data, entomological data, and infection data. The following study questions and objective are addressed.

1.6 Study questions and objectives

1.6.1 Study questions

1. To what extent does weather at the micro scale level affect malaria transmission among under five children (U5s) in a holoendemic area?
2. Can malaria be predicted at local scale using weather parameters as a driving force?

1.6.2 Main objective

To develop and validate a dynamic model based on weather parameters to locally predict the risk of malaria transmission and forecast outbreaks among U5s in a holo-endemic area of Africa.

1.6.3 Specific objectives

1. To assess the incidence of *P. falciparum* infection and clinical malaria among U5s in four different ecological settings in a holoendemic area, north-west Burkina Faso.
2. To determine the effect of temperature, rainfall and relative humidity on *P. falciparum* infection risk among U5s in a holoendemic area, north-west Burkina Faso
3. To determine the impact of temperature, rainfall on mosquitoes population dynamics in a holo-endemic area, north-west Burkina Faso
4. To assess the *P. falciparum* seasonal transmission pressure among U5s in a holo-endemic area, north-west Burkina Faso.
5. To develop and validate a dynamic weather-based model of predicting malaria transmission risk.
6. To address the study question and objective we have developed a conceptual framework.

1.7 Conceptual framework

The malaria transmission model combines the human host and the vector host models (Figure 1.10). Both of them can be compartmentalised into susceptible, infected and infectious groups and they are linked by the mosquito blood meal. Susceptible (H_1) individuals move to the infected group (H_2) after an infectious mosquito bite. During the blood meal, the mosquito injects the parasite into the humans' blood. The likelihood of the person moving from the susceptible to the infected compartment depends on the prevention measures taken for protection against mosquitoes bites. An infected person develops the parasite and moves to the stage of infectious (H_3) depending on prophylaxis and immune status. If proper

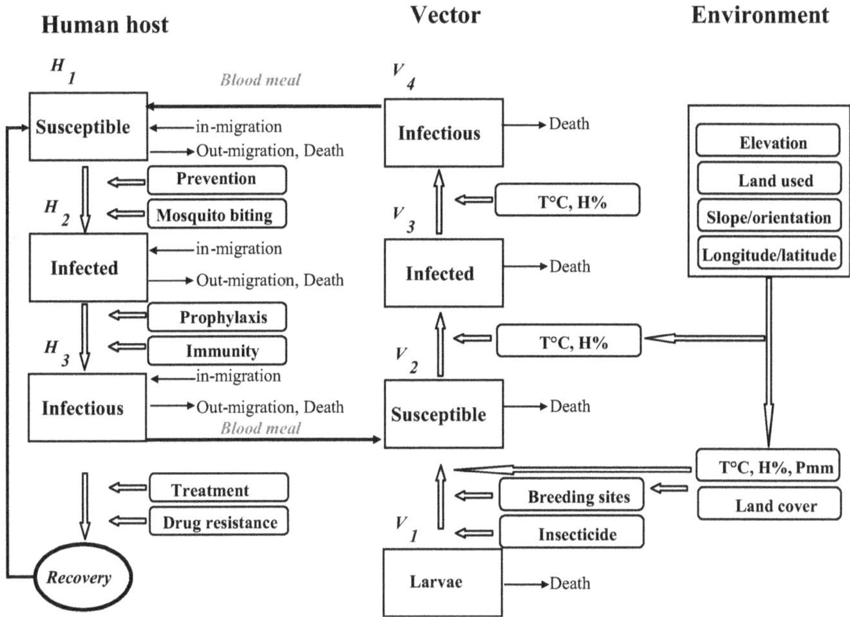

Figure 1.10 Conceptual model for malaria transmission

treatment is given, the person will recover and become susceptible again after the washout period of the treatment.

A susceptible (V_2) mosquito is a result of the development from the larvae (V_1) stage to an adult mosquito. This process is dependent on the environment. Some external conditions need to be fulfilled for the process to be completed. The first condition is presence of suitable breeding sites. The cycle takes an average of ten days and this means the microclimate condition of the breeding site have to be optimal for at least this period otherwise the development process will not be complete. The second condition is the temperature. The mosquito becomes infected (V_3) after a blood meal from an infectious human. It will then develop the parasite and become infectious (V_4). The time delay between the infected and infectious stage of the mosquito largely depends on the ambient temperature as already extensively discussed (section 1.3.3.1).

Chapter 2
Population, Material and Methods

2.1 Study design

To develop the models based on field data, a population-based prospective cohort study was conducted. A cohort of 867 children aged between 6 and 59 months were recruited through random selection of their households from three villages (Goni, Cissé and Kodougou) and Nouna town. These children were followed for 12 months (01.12.2003–30.11.2004) over one dry and one rainy season for active parasite detection. The longitudinal study started and ended with a cross-sectional survey. In addition, we prospectively assessed exposure variables such as land cover, meteorological factors (temperature, rainfall, and relative humidity) and mosquito biting variable by field-based data collection and satellite imagery. A detailed description of each survey is given in the following section.

2.2 Study sites

The study took place in Nouna town and the villages of Cissé, Goni and Kodougou. These four sites are part of the Nouna Demographic Surveillance Systems area, which is located in Kossi province in the North-Western part of Burkina Faso (latitudes 12°49' and 12°96' north and between longitudes 3°53' and 4°06' west), Figure 2.1. The climate is hot with a short rainy season (June–September, total annual rain varying between 600 and 900 mm). The other months are dry without any rainfall. The average annual temperature is about 29°C with wide variation during the year. The hottest month is April with average temperature of 34°C and the coldest is January with an average of 28°C. The temperature variation is more evident when monthly minima and maxima averages are compared. The vegetation is mainly dry savannah comprised of scattered short trees. More dense vegetation is found near the two main rivers (*Le Mouhoun* and *Le Sourou*). The population is composed of mainly farmers and cattle herders. Farming (mostly subsistence crops) is limited to the rainy season, except for the villages neighbouring the rivers, where the permanent presence of water allows dry season farming (mainly vegetables).

The choice of Nouna DSS area as a study site was justified by several factors. First is it a high malaria endemic area with high seasonal variation of malaria transmission. Malaria is the major cause of death among U5s. Second, the DSS provides accurate regularly updated information on the population characteristics. 60,000 individuals are being followed up since 1992 by continuous registration

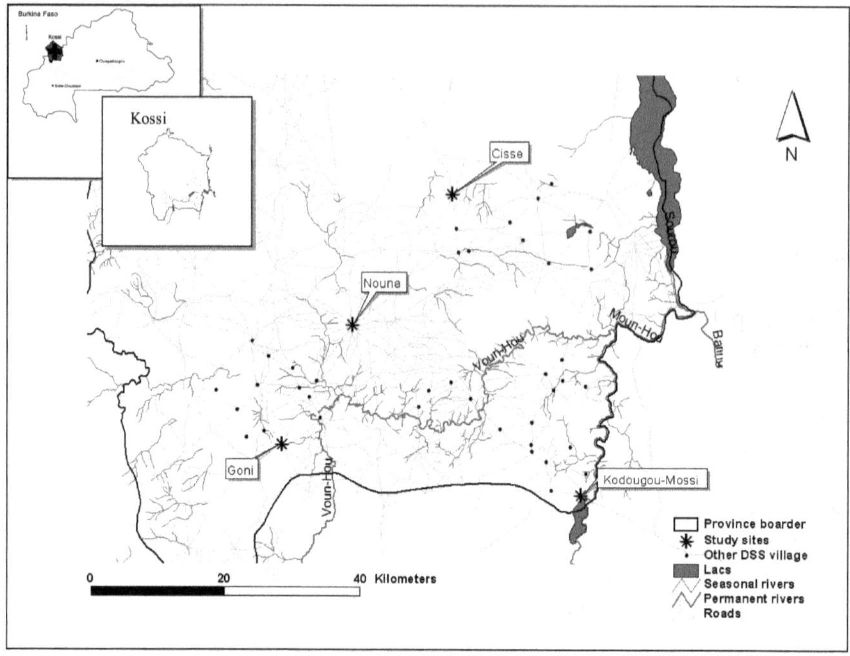

Figure 2.1 Location of the study sites

of their vital events (birth, death, immigration and emigration) providing a unique database (Ye et al. 2001). The study participants were recruited randomly from this database, without having to conduct a baseline survey. Third, the DSS database is linked to a GIS which is comprised of a digital map georeference of all the households within the DSS area. Fourth, the CRSN multidisciplinary research capacity and facilities offered indispensable support for the study. The biological and entomological laboratories capacities were used for parasite detection and mosquitoes processing. Finally, the strong collaboration of the CRSN and the Health District made setting up an early treatment and referral system possible.

2.3 Malaria infection survey

2.3.1 Sampling procedure

2.3.1.1 Selection of study sites The four sites (Nouna, Goni and Kodougou), were 19–44 km from each other (see Figure 2.1) and were chosen on purpose to represent the different ecological and human settings in the region. Nouna is a semi-urban area with 25,000 inhabitants while the other three sites are rural villages with a population of 980, 3,170 and 1,308 respectively Cissé, Goni and

Kodougou. Nouna is located in a plain and is flooded during the rainy season. Kodougou is a village by a perennial river, while the villages of Goni and Cissé are near a rice field and a forest reserve respectively. Different ecological settings are expected to support different malaria transmission dynamics. Digital weather stations, measuring temperature, relative humidity and rainfall were located in each of the study sites except Goni, for which it was located five kilometres away in the neighbouring village of Toni. These two villages share the same ecological setting. Toni was initially selected as a study site, but was reconsidered to avoid interference with another malaria research project. The project was an intervention study evaluating home-based treatment of malaria by mothers. In this project, the drugs provided were subsidised, but had to be bought by mothers. In our project, all children were to be treated free. Clearly the two studies were not compatible. This would have had an important impact on the trial project.

2.3.1.2 Sample size estimation The sample size was calculated to detect a difference of a least 10% prevalence of *P. falciparum* infection between the four ecological settings, with 80% power and significance of 5%. Calculations were done in StatCalc – Epi Info. The samples size calculation (for cohort study) option of Epi Info 2002 was used to estimate the number of children required. The probability of reflecting the true difference between the site if there is any was set to 95% or α=5%, the probability of detecting the significant difference, or power was set to 80%. Expected prevalence of malaria in the low prevalence sites was assumed to be 35% (based on unpublished data), with risk ratio (malaria infection) of 1.30. The number of children in each site was set to be equal, with a ratio between exposed and unexposed equal to 1. This gave a sample size of 720 children. To keep the power over the follow up time, we increased the sample size to account for refusal, inability to take part in or failure to identify the participant from the DSS (10%), and loss to follow up (15%). In total 180 children were added to 720, to give a final sample of 900 (225 children per site).

2.3.1.3 Selection of study participants Children in each site were selected through their household (cluster) (Figure 2.2). A list of household with children fulfilling the age criteria (6–59 months) was drawn up for each site from the DSS database. The list was sorted alphabetically using the name of the head of household. A systematic sampling procedure was used to select the household. The sampling interval was calculated and the starting point selected from a list of random numbers. The sampling interval was calculated as follows: Let H be the total number of households with at least one 6–59 months old child in the site, N the total number of children (6–59 months) in the site, n the sample size in the site ($n=225$), h the total number of households needed to reach n and a the average number of children in a household:

$$\left(a = \frac{N}{H}\right),$$

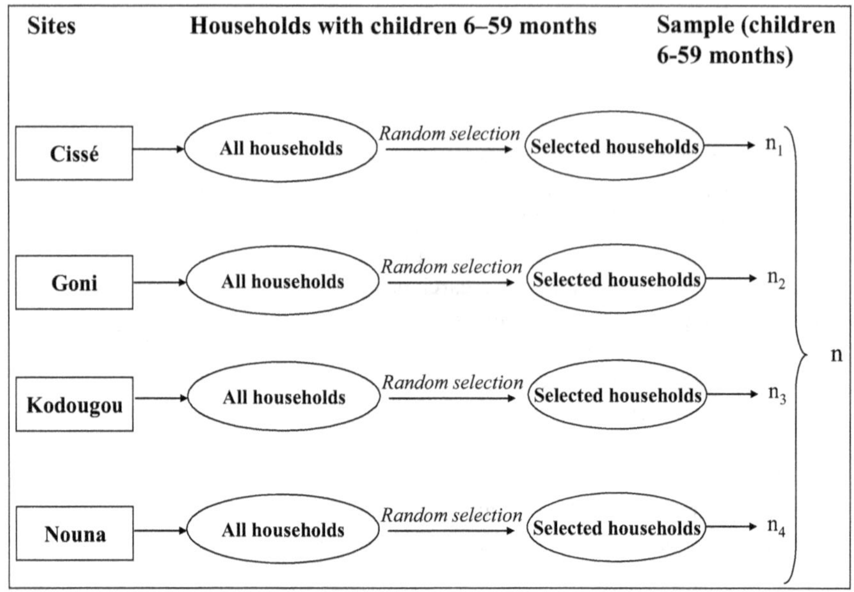

Figure 2.2 Sampling procedure

then $h = \frac{a}{n}$

and the sampling interval $i = \frac{H}{h}$

rounded off to the nearest integer (Table 2.1).

Table 2.1 Definition of sampling interval for the four villages

	Sites				
	Cissé	Goni	Kodougou	Nouna	Total
H	84	260	89	1,601	2,034
N	192	540	217	2,778	3,727
$A = N/H$	2.28	2.07	2.43	1.73	1.83
SD	1.41	1.31	2.16	1.02	1.19
Maximum children/ household	7	9	10	9	10
$h = \frac{a}{n}$	99	109	93	130	
$i = \frac{H}{h}$	-	2	-	12	

There was no need for sampling for Cissé and Kodougou where the total number of children was below 225; therefore, all the children were selected. To reach 900 children, we over sampled in Goni and Nouna. Initially children selected were visited at home for identification and to seek informed consent (Annex 2) for their participation from their parent or legal guardian. Out of 900 children initially selected, 867 were successfully identified. 33 children were either unknown (10) or had emigrated (23) to another village.

2.3.2 Data collection

2.3.2.1 Cross-sectional survey Two cross-sectional surveys were conducted at the beginning (14–18.11.2003) and the end (29.11–5.12.04) of the follow-up to assess the prevalence of *P. falciparum* infection among participants. While in the first one we only tested for parasites in febrile children, in the second all participants were tested. The field and laboratory procedures in both cases were identical. A mobile team including one physician, one nurse, two laboratory technicians and five interviewers visited each site. Mothers were asked to bring their children to a meeting point identified by the village chief. Children were first identified by preprinted questionnaire (Annex 3) and screened for fever using digital axillary thermometers. Febrile (body temperature >=37.5°C) children were physically examined, including weight measurement and spleen palpation and then treated with Chloroquine (25mg/kg weight during three days: day 1: 10mg/kg, single intake; day 2: 10mg/kg, single intake; day 3: 5mg/kg) and Paracetamol. Severely sick children were referred, at the cost of the project to the nearest health centre for treatment. After the clinical examination, a blood sample was obtained by finger prick method. A thick and thin blood slides were prepared; the slides were coded and carefully stored in boxes. The blood slides were later stained with Giemsa and read by microscope for parasite count in the CRSN laboratory. Parasite density was estimated by counting 100 fields and equating this to 0.25µl of blood. In addition, mothers were asked about the use of mosquito nets and antimalaria drugs in the previous week.

All data, including physical examination, net and antimalaria drug use, and laboratory test results were recorded on forms (Annex 3).

2.3.2.2 Longitudinal survey (active case detection) Five interviewers were trained for a week on body temperature measurement, finger prick, and thin and thick slide preparation procedures. In addition, they were trained on malaria symptoms identification and administration of first line treatment. One interviewer was allocated to each of the sites, while the fifth was used as a backup. He would immediately take over whenever one of the permanent interviewers was sick or unavailable for any other reason, so the follow-up was uninterrupted.

Interviewers were permanently based in the sites and were equipped with all required materials, such as slides, lancets, medical alcohol, cotton wool, gloves, slide storage boxes, digital thermometers and drugs for first line treatment (Chloroquine and Paracetamol). They were visited every week by a field supervisor and materials were supplied if necessary. In each site, children were visited every week at home. As the aim was to assess the impact of weather conditions on malaria infection, we made sure the visits were synchronised in all the four sites. All the children were seen in the first three days of the week according to a predefined schedule (Annex 4). Visiting children at different times would have made the comparison difficult since the weather may change. Interviewers were given bicycles for easy travel between households.

At each visit, body temperature was measured, blood sample (finger prick) taken for febrile children (axillary temperature => 37.5) and presumptive treatment given as in the cross-sectional survey. The mothers were also asked about bednet use. The questions was consistently asked in the following way, "After my last visit, has your child been sleeping under a mosquito net every night? If yes, which net? Impregnated or not?" All data were reported in a form (Annex 5). The forms contained preprinted data (identification, sex, date of birth ...) of the child. The identification of the blood slide, if any, was also reported in this form. This identification number was composed of the child identification number and the number of visit. In case of absence of the children during the visit, detailed information of the reason, destination and duration of the absence were recorded on a specific form (Annex 6).

Children under treatment were monitored at home (body temperature) every day, and additional information reported (Annex 7). In case of no improvement, the child was referred to the nearest Health Centre, or the District referral hospital. All medical and related costs were covered by the project.

Stored blood slides were collected by the field supervisor at each of his visits and transported to the CRSN laboratory. There, the slides were stained with Giemsa and read for parasite count. Each slide was read twice by different laboratory technicians to confirm the result. In case of conflict, the biologist was involved for the third reading. In such cases only the biologist's reading was considered. This happened in only 2% of the slides, suggesting little inter-reader variability. Laboratory results were reported on a specific form (Annex 8) to ease data entry.

The primary outcome measured was a new episode of *P. falciparum* infection, defined as axillary temperature => 37.5°C plus positive parasite test. The secondary outcome was a malaria episode defined as fever plus at least 5,000 parasites/µl. This case definition was similar to Müller et al. (2001, 2003). The use of these two outcomes was justified because in endemic areas, due to immunity, the presence of parasites does not necessarily lead to clinical malaria. In addition, both asymptomatic and symptomatic cases contribute to the transmission process.

2.3.2.3 Household survey This survey was conducted in the first week of the month. The aim was to collect data on households characteristics (discussed in the introduction) which were likely to have an impact on malaria transmission and confound the weather and land cover effects. A month was proper since such factors are unlikely to vary at a shorter interval. The survey was always conducted by the same interviewers (section 2.3.2.2) in the household of the children under survey. It consisted of a structured interview with the head of household and individual members when necessary (history of malaria episodes and use of antimalaria medicine) using a specific questionnaire (Annex 9). The questionnaire was comprised of three sections. Section one was about the history of malaria in the household. All members were asked (mother for children under 15 years) about their history of malaria and treatment in the preceding month. The reference date was the last visit of the interviewer. Whenever any treatment was reported, the drug, dosage and duration of treatment was asked for. The second section concerned the use of mosquito nets in the household. The head of household was asked about the number of mosquito nets in his household and the type (impregnated or not). Section three was about housing conditions: the material used for the wall (mud block, grass, stone, or cement bricks) and the roof (Iron sheet, mud or grass). Since in this area, a typical household compound is comprised of several houses, the house where the child participant sleeps was considered. The conditions in the surrounding area of the household (30 metres radius), such as presence of animals, well or potential mosquito breeding site were recorded. All answers were cross checked by observation.

2.4 Entomological survey

Sampling of mosquitoes was performed from December 2003 to November 2004. Three conventional methods for field mosquito sampling were used: Light Trap Capture (LTC), Human Land Capture (HLC) and Pyrethrum Spray Capture (PSC). These three methods were complementary. Using HLC with simultaneous indoor and outdoor catchers enabled us to identify the proportion of *endophily* and *exophily* species. HLC is the most accurate method to estimate the vector aggressiveness and human biting rate. However, young and hungry mosquitoes are more likely to be caught. It also poses ethical issues since human attendants have to be exposed to malaria infection risk and other mosquito-borne diseases. LTC is the safest method for humans and the most commonly used to estimate mosquito abundance and biting rates. It can be calibrated with the HLC and provides a more balanced sample of mosquito species distribution. PSC is designed to sample indoor fed mosquitoes and is only suitable for *endophagic* (vector feeding and resting indoor) vector. However, it gives an estimate of the number of *anthropophilic* (preference for feeding on humans or human blood index) and *zoophilic* (preference for feeding on animals) vectors.

2.4.1 Selection of sampling houses

Mosquito captures were performed in each of the four study sites. To avoid interference, different households were selected for each of the mosquito sampling methods. Households were randomly selected and a capture schedule developed for the whole study period (Annex 10). The schedule indicated the selected household, the type of capture to be performed and the exact dates. The different methods were performed at different time, but four households were used (Table 2.2).

Table 2.2 Mosquitoes capture schedule

Captures	Months	Number of houses per month	Number of nights per month
LTC	Monthly	4	2
HLC	January, March, May, July, August, September, October	4	2
PSC	August, September, October	4	3

Four households were selected to have a fair geographical distribution of the sampling points. They were assumed to cover the different conditions in the village. The number of nights was two, assuming, for each month, the abundance of mosquitoes will not be significantly different between consecutive nights. Two night captures per month were sufficient to reduce sampling bias because of weather variation, such as rainfall, cloud cover, or moonlight. A bright moonlight gives an impression of daylight to mosquitoes and therefore they may remain hidden.

2.4.2 Mosquito sampling

2.4.2.1 Light Trap Capture (LTC) Centre for disease Control (CDC) light traps (Model 512; John W. Hock Company, Gainesville, Florida, USA) were used to capture mosquitoes indoors. Trained entomological fieldworkers set up the light traps fitted with incandescent bulbs close to the child sleeping under an untreated mosquito net (Figure 2.3a). In case the child was using a treated net, the parents were asked for consent to replace it with a non-treated one just for the two consecutive nights of capture. The Light traps operated from 18.00 to 06.00 hours and mosquitoes caught were emptied in the morning (Figure 2.3b). Mosquitoes were later sorted and counted and the numbers reported (Annex 11). Additional information on the sampling place was collected using a form (Annex 12). This form included individual characteristics of the person under the net and other persons in the house. It also included the type of protection against mosquitoes

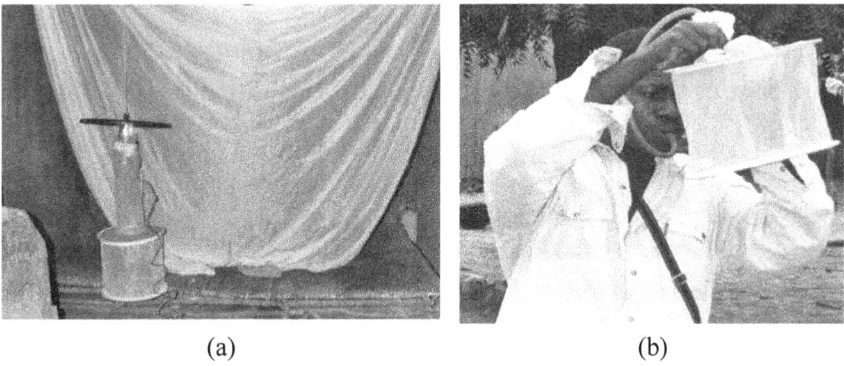

(a) (b)

Figure 2.3 (a) CDC light trap set by a volunteer under mosquito net, (b) Entomological fieldworker extracting the mosquitoes caught from the trap

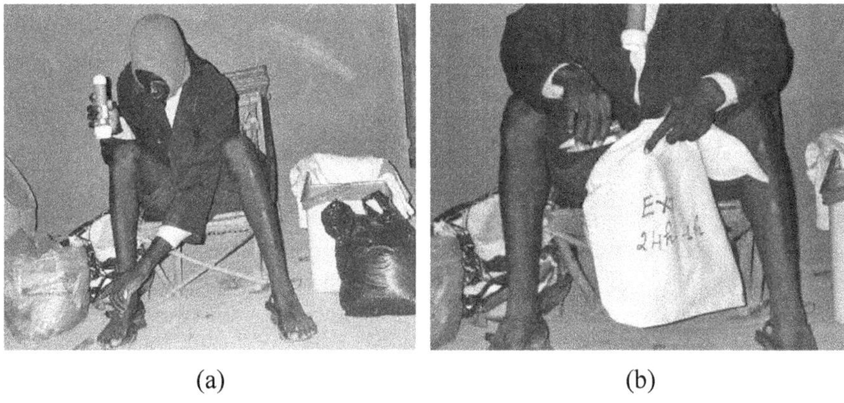

(a) (b)

Figure 2.4 (a) volunteer catching mosquitoes with a tube, (b) Storing mosquitoes caught

used, the presence of animal in the compound and the status of the trap in the morning (whether still on or not), and finally, the weather (rainfall, or windy).

2.4.2.2 Human Land Capture (HLC) HLC was performed in and outdoors every two months during the dry season (December, February, April, June) and every month during the rainy season (July, August, September and October). It consisted of two adults equipped with a watch, one sitting inside an uninhabited house and the other outside, and collecting mosquitoes that landed on their exposed legs using torchlight and test tubes (Figure 2.4a). The pairs of collectors were replaced after six hours to avoid sampling bias because of impaired performance. Collections took place from 18.00 to 06.00 hours. Mosquitoes caught were stored in separate bags according to the times of capture (Figure 2.4b). For example a mosquito caught by a person sitting outside between 24h00 and 01h00 was stored in the bag labelled "Ex 24h–01h00" (meaning outdoor capture from 24h00–01h00).

2.4.2.3 Pyrethrum Spray Capture (PSC) It was performed for three consecutive nights only during the high transmission period (August, September and October 2004). In each site, four households (different from HLC and LTC houses) were randomly selected. At 06:00 am, two entomological fieldworkers used white cloth sheets to cover every floor area inside the selected houses. The doors and windows were closed, and the inside was sprayed with insecticide for about one minute. After ten minutes, the knocked out mosquitoes on the white sheets were collected. Inhabitants of selected house were informed the day before. In total 144 captures were performed on nine different days. Data on housing conditions which were likely to influence the sampling were also collected using forms (Annex 13). Housing conditions data comprised house's location, number of person who has slept in the house that night, use of bednet (impregnated or not), insecticide's use, biomass burning the previous night, presence of animal in the house or compound.

2.4.2.4 Mosquito processing Mosquitoes caught each night were transported to the laboratory in a cold-box. Specimens were counted and sorted by species. LT, HLT and PSC mosquitoes were classified into "unfed", "partly fed", "fully fed", "semi-gravid" or "gravid", by external inspection (LT and PSC) or dissection (HLT). The ovaries of unfed HLT mosquitoes were dissected on a slide to check for parity by observation, using microscopy, of the ovarian tracheoles (Detinova 1963). *Nulliparous* mosquitoes (females which have not yet oviposited) had their ovaries covered with tightly coiled tracheole skeins, whereas in parous female (females which had laid one or more batches of eggs) the skeins were unravelled (Gilles and Warrell 1993). The results of the dissection were reported on a form. (Annex 14). All mosquitoes were stored in Eppendorf® tubes with silica gel, separated from mosquitoes by cotton wool. Samples were labelled and stored in a freezer for further use.

2.5 Weather data

Weather data were measured on the ground using Digital Dataloggers (THIES Datalogger, MeteoLOG TDL 14) installed in each of the four sites (Nouna, Kodougou, Cissé, Toni for Goni as mentioned above). The stations were set to measure mosquito feeding site conditions, and were therefore installed by the village side (average distance of 100 metres). A meteorological unit was composed of three sensors (temperature, humidity and rainfall). Ambient temperature and

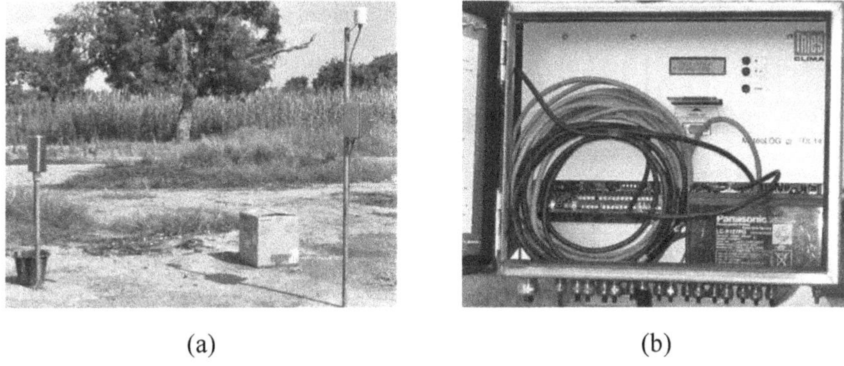

(a) (b)

Figure 2.5 (a) Weather unit in Kodougou village, (b) data loggers

humidity sensor were combined in one single unit, while the rainfall sensor was separate (Figure 2.5)

Following World Meteorological Organization standards, the temperature and humidity sensor was set 2.5 metres above the ground and the rainfall one at 1.5 metres. The data loggers were set on 10-second measurements cycles and values were recorded automatically every 10 minutes. For ambient temperature, rainfall and relative humidity, the mean of the 10-second cycles was recorded every 10 minutes and for rainfall the sum of the 10-second values was recorded.

Power for the Dataloggers was supplied by a rechargeable battery, which could last for about one and half months. To ensure security and uninterrupted measurement, local persons were recruited in each site. Their task was to look after the unit and immediately tell the meteorological supervisor (based in Nouna), if there was any problem. Every month, the Meteorological supervisor visited the site and the data were downloaded from the data logger to a memory card and later transferred into a weather database at the CRSN. Daily average temperature, relative humidity and total rainfall were then calculated.

The summary of data collected and time-frame is given in Figure 2.6.

2.6 Data processing

2.6.1 Data entry and cleaning

Malaria, mosquito and weather data were entered continuously into a relational database (Figure 2.7) in Microsoft Access XP®. The relational model allowed follow-up data from different factors to be entered. To minimise entry mistakes, the data entry screen was similar to the data collection forms. We included consistency checks at data entry. One full-time data entry clerk was in charge of entering the data.

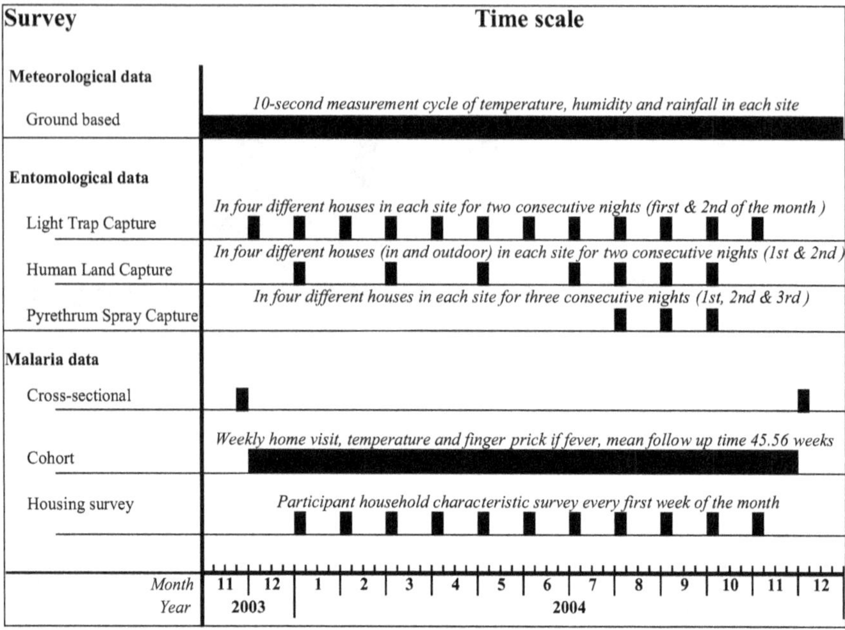

Figure 2.6 Schematic representation of the study design and timetable

2.6.2 Quality control

Quality control was preformed at the field and at data entry levels. For each survey, a field supervisor was assigned. Their tasks consisted of visiting the fieldworkers in the fields and checking the filled forms before sending them for data entry. Any problem they detected was reported to the fieldworkers for correction. Parasitological survey fieldworkers were visited by a physician and biologist every two months for supervision.

At the data entry level, a data entry supervisor checked randomly 5% of data entered each day. The critical proportion of error was set to the 5% level. Data were to be re-entered if the proportion of mistakes was above 5%. However, this never occurred. Forms with inconsistent information were sent back to the field team for correction. Since the data were entered parallel with the data collections, correction and feedback were possible.

2.6.3 Final data cleaning

The data cleaning process consisted of eliminating the inconsistent values that were not identified through the quality control step. Missing values were also coded. We used MS Access® query to produce frequency tables and detect inconsistencies if any. Most of inconsistencies were corrected by going back to original forms.

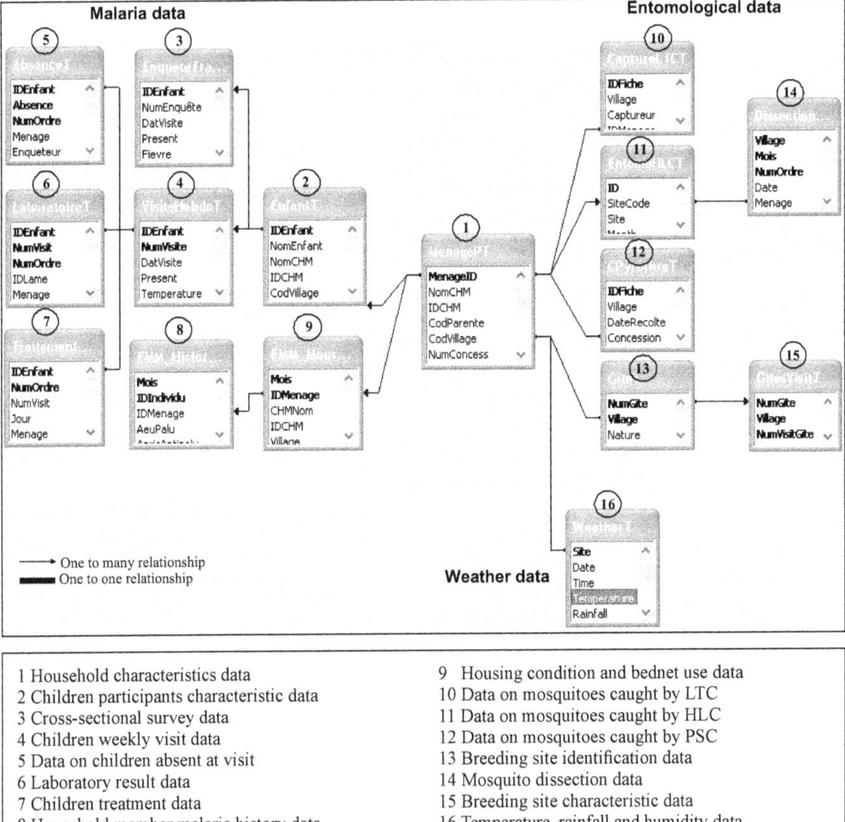

Figure 2.7 Relational data base architecture

Those few which could not be traced were simply coded as missing values. Final tables containing clean data were exported to statistical package for analysis.

2.7 Data analysis

2.7.1 Weather data

For each site, daily temperatures (mean, minimum and maximum), total rainfall/ day and relative humidity were calculated using average function for temperature and humidity, and sum function for rainfall. For temperature and humidity, the 10-minute values were summed up and divided by the number of measurements in a day (144) to get the daily average. For rainfall it was the cumulative values of every 10 minutes that gave the total rainfall in the day. Using similar procedures, the weekly and monthly values for each parameter were calculated from daily values (Table 2.3). All the calculations were done in MS Excel XP® spreadsheet.

Table 2.3 Calculation methods for meteorological indicators

Parameters	Periods				
	10 minutes	**Daily**	**Weekly**	**Months**	**Year**
Temperature					
Mean	Recorded, $\frac{\sum of 10 \sec onds values}{60}$	Calculated, $\frac{\sum of 10 mn values}{144}$	Calculated, $\frac{\sum of 7 days values}{7}$	Calculated, $\frac{\sum of month day values}{month days}$	Calculated, $\frac{\sum of month values}{12}$
Mini		Minimum value of 10 mn values	Calculated, $\frac{\sum of \min day values}{7}$	Calculated, $\frac{\sum of \min day values}{month days}$	Calculated, $\frac{\sum of \min month values}{12}$
Maxi		Maximum value of 10 mn values	Calculated, $\frac{\sum of \max day values}{7}$	Calculated, $\frac{\sum of \max day values}{month days}$	Calculated, $\frac{\sum of \max month values}{12}$
Relative Humidity	Recorded, $\frac{\sum of 10 \sec onds values}{60}$	Calculated, $\frac{\sum of 10 mn values}{144}$	Calculated, $\frac{\sum of 7 days values}{7}$	Calculated, $\frac{\sum of month day values}{month days}$	Calculated, $\frac{\sum of month values}{12}$
Rainfall	Recorded, ∑ of 10 second value	Calculated, ∑ of 10 mn value	Calculated, ∑ of 7 mn value	Calculated, ∑ of month days value	Calculated, ∑ of 12 months value

The mosquito development process is heavily affected by weather variation. To compare the variation of weather between the sites, for temperature and relative humidity, the weekly, monthly and yearly standard deviations were calculated in each site.

2.7.2 Mosquito data

2.7.2.1 Calculation of mosquito abundance Monthly mosquito abundance for each site was calculated by summing-up the number of mosquitoes caught from the four capture points according to the different species and type of capture. Only the malaria vectors were broken down to subspecies (*An. gambiae, An. funestus, An nili*). Focus was on *An. gambiae* which is the main malaria vector in this region.

2.7.2.2 Estimation of physiological age of An. gambiae population The age structure of *An. gambiae* population was assessed by calculating the proportion of *multiparous*, female which was expressed by the fraction of old *An. gambiae* having laid eggs at least once. This is the most dangerous vector population. In contrast, *nulliparous* are young and newly emerged mosquitoes. A high fraction of *nulliparous* will mean young populations. The calculation was done on the HLT mosquitoes for each site and only using the dissected unfed *An. gambiae*.

2.7.2.3 Estimation of human biting rate and EIR Indoor human biting rates were calculated for each month and site. As expressed by Macdonald (1957), it indicates the number of bites per person per night (*ma*). It was calculated as follows: Human biting rate: $ma = Bs/P\ /n$, where, *Bs* is the number of *An. gambiae* caught indoor by HLT during the monthly two night-captures, *P* the number of persons involved in the capture, which was 8 per month and site, and *n* the total number of night when the capture took place (2 nights). Since we did not test for human blood index (proportion of *An.* tested positive for human blood), we have assumed that all the mosquitoes were *anthropophiles* (feed on human).

The estimation of the EIR required the mosquitoes to be tested by ELISA for sporozoite detection (infectious mosquito). As this was not possible, we used the proportion of *parous* mosquitoes. These are mosquitoes which have oviposited at least once and are likely to be infectious. The number of *parous* mosquitoes was then divided by the number of persons involved in the human capture and divided by the number of days. This resulted in the number of infected bites received per person per night. The monthly and yearly rates were then calculated by simply multiplying the daily rate by 30 and 365.25 days respectively.

2.7.2.4 Comparison of HLC and LTC As the HLC was not performed every month, because of reasons already mentioned, we tested whether LTC could be an alternative for those months when HLC data were not available. We calculated the correlation coefficient (r^2), comparing for each site indoor HLC *An. gambiae* to LTC. An estimate of $r^2>0.75$ was set as an acceptable correlation suggesting the methods were comparable and either method could be used.

2.7.2.5 Estimation of An. gambiae mortality and vectorial capacity *An. gambiae* generation mortality (*k-value*) was calculated monthly for each site. It expressed the number of vectors surviving from the egg stage to the adult stage. Monthly number of vector was transformed into natural logarithm plus 1. We assumed the maximum number of eggs oviposited (fertility) by individual mosquitoes was on average *m*=100 eggs (Depinay et al. 2004, Lyimo and Takken 1993, Takken et al. 1998). *k value* was calculated as follows:

> log(potential eggs/month 1)=log(adults+1/month 1)+log(maximum individual fertility), and $K_{month\ 1}$ =log (potential eggs/month 1)-log(adults+1/month 2). (Rogers 1983) The monthly mortality rate (*M*) could be calculated by the following formula: $M = 1 - 10^{-kvalue}$

The Vectorial capacity (expected inoculations of human per infective case per time unit) was calculated monthly and for each site using Macdonald's (1957) formula.

$$\frac{ma^2p^n}{-\ln p},$$

where *a* is the mosquito feeding frequency, *m* the human blood index, *p* the daily mosquito population survival probability and *n* the sporogonic cycle. Again here some assumptions have to be made. One such assumption is that mosquitoes are feeding on infectious human and every bite will cause a vector infection. The daily survival probability was calculated as followed:

$$p = 10^{-monthkvalue/d},$$

where *d* is the number of days in the month.

The sporogonic duration was calculated using Detivova's (1962) formula 111/T°C-18, where T°C is the monthly mean temperature in degree Celsius.

2.7.3 Infection data

2.7.3.1 Descriptive analysis For each site, the monthly incidence rate (IR) per 1,000 for the total cohort was calculated. This was done by first calculating the monthly person-time, which is the total number of days under observation divided by the number of days in the given months, or in the year for person years. Since the observation was done every week, a child present at the visit was assumed to have contributed seven days. A child seen at all the 52 visits of the study period was assumed to have contributed 365 days/365.35, or one person year. The person time was then used as a denominator to calculate the incidence rate. It was expressed as the total number of new cases divided by the person-time. We calculated the incidence for two outcomes. The first was the *P. falciparum* infection, which was defined as a fever plus a parasite positive slide. The second was the clinical malaria case, defined as fever plus *P. falciparum* density >=5000µl.

2.7.3.2 Multilevel modelling, comparing infection risk by site A multilevel statistical modelling (logistic regression binary response) approach was used to assess the influence of place of residence on the odds of being *P. falciparum* infection positive. Nouna, as an urban site was used as a reference. The rationale of using the multilevel approach was derived from the hierarchical structure of the data. Repeated measurements (level 1) were taken from children (level 2) who were clustered in a household (level 3). Since measures were taken for the same individual several times they were likely to be autocorrelated. In addition, within a household the risk of malaria is likely to be similar for members because they share the same socio-economic and housing conditions which were not measured in the study. Using simple regression would have implied that observation were indeed interdependent in the same individual and within the same household. We would therefore have violated the basic assumption of independence of observation. Ignoring this fact would have led to biased estimates of parameters.

Table 2.4 List and description of variables included in the models

Factors	Variable	Description	Type	Value
Outcome	*P. falciparum* infection	Fever + slide test positive presence of parasite	Binary	0=No 1=Yes
	P. falciparum malaria	Fever + parasite density >=5000	Binary	0=No 1=Yes
Residence	Site	Site of residence of the child	Categorical	1=Nouna (ref) 2=Cissé 3=Goni 4=Kodougou
Individual characteristics	Sex	Sex of the child	Binary	0=Male (ref) 1=Female
	Age	Age group in month	Categorical	0=< 12 1=12–23 2=24–35 3=36–47 4=48+(ref)
	Ethnic	Ethnic group to which the child belonged	Categorical	1=Peulh (ref) 2=Mossi 3=Marka 4=Bwaba 5=Samo 6=other
Prevention	Net use	Did the child sleep under the mosquito net since the last visit?	Binary	0=No (ref) 1=Yes
	Treated	Received treatment in the previous visit	Binary	0=No (ref) 1=Yes
	NbrNetHHS	Ratio, number of mosquito net and number of persons in the household	Binary	0= ratio<1 (ref) 1=ratio>1

Table 2.4 *continued*

Factors	Variable	Description	Type	Value
Housing conditions	Wall	Type of material the house is made of where the child usually sleeps	Binary	0=not concrete (ref), 1=Concrete
	Roof	Type of material the roof of the house is made of where the child usually sleeps	Categorical	1=Iron sheet (ref), 2=Mud, 3=Gras
	Animal	Presence of animal enclosure within 30 meters radius of the household	Binary	0=No (ref), 1=Yes
	Breeding	Presence of open water body	Binary	0=No (ref), 1=Yes
	Well	Presence of well	Binary	0=No (ref), 1=Yes
	Farm	Presence of farm	Binary	0=not farm (ref), 1=Farm
Climate	Season	Dry season= November to May, Rainy season= June to September	Binary	0=Dry season 1=Rainy season

ref = reference categories

To enable comparison between the estimate of the conventional logistic regression (single level) and the ones from the multilevel model with random intercepts, both models were run. The variables described in Table 2.4 were included in both models. Since backward elimination of the non significant variables did not change the estimates we decided to keep all variables in the final model.

1. Conventional logistic regression model
The model was built as following:

$$
\begin{aligned}
\log it(\pi_i) = \; & \beta_0 + \beta_1 Site\_Cisse_i + \beta_2 Site\_Goni_i + \beta_3 Site\_Kodougou_i + \beta_4 Sex\_Female_i \\
& + \beta_5 Age\_<12_i + \beta_6 Age\_12-23_i + \beta_7 Age\_24_i - 35 + \beta_8 Age\_36-47_i \\
& + \beta_9 Ethnic\_Mossi_i + \beta_{10} Ethnic\_Marka_i + \beta_{11} Ethnic\_Bwaba_i + \beta_{12} Ethnic\_Samo_i \\
& + \beta_{13} Ethnic\_other_i + \beta_{14} Netused\_Yes_i + \beta_{15} Wall\_Concret_i + \beta_{16} Roof\_Mud_i \\
& + \beta_{17} Roof\_Grass_i + \beta_{18} Well\_Yes_i + \beta_{19} Animal\_Yes_i + \beta_{20} Breedingsite\_Yes_i \\
& + \beta_{21} NbrNetHHS_i + \beta_{22} Season\_Rainy_i
\end{aligned}
$$

Where π_i is the predicted probability of being *P. falciparum* infection or clinical malaria positive of the *i*th child. The odds of the same child will be

$$\frac{\pi_i}{1-\pi_i},$$

β_0 the intercept, and $\beta_1 \dots \beta_{26}$ the regression coefficients of the independent variables (name following each coefficient). The odds ratio associated with *Site_Cissé* I compared to Nouna (reference) is the exponential of β_1 (OR $_{Site\_Cissé}$ =exp(β_1)). The significance of the OR was assessed using 95% confidence intervals (CI). An estimate with a CI not including one expressed significant odds of the variable on the outcomes compared to the reference group.

2. Multilevel model (three levels random intercept)
This model contained the same covariates as in the conventional one. Three levels of the data structure were defined. The level one is the weekly repeated measurements for *P. falciparum* infection (52 times) on one individual child. The second level is the individual child belonging to household which is the third level. Households are distributed among the four sites. The model was defined as follows:

$$
\begin{aligned}
\log it(\pi_{ijk}) = \; & \beta_{0jk} + \beta_1 Site\_Cisse_{ijk} + \beta_2 Site\_Goni_{ijk} + \beta_3 Site\_Kodougou_{ijk} \\
& + \beta_4 Sex\_Female_{ijk} + \beta_5 Age\_<12_{ijk} + \beta_6 Age\_12-23_{ijk} \\
& + \beta_7 Age\_24_{ijk} - 35 + \beta_8 Age\_36-47_{ijk} + \beta_9 Ethnic\_Mossi_{ijk} \\
& + \beta_{10} Ethnic\_Marka_{ijk} + \beta_{11} Ethnic\_Bwaba_{ijk} + \beta_{12} Ethnic\_Samo_{ijk} \\
& + \beta_{13} Ethnic\_other_{ijk} + \beta_{14} Netused\_Yes_{ijk} + \beta_{15} Wall\_Concret_{ijk} \\
& + \beta_{16} Roof\_Mud_{ijk} + \beta_{17} Roof\_Grass_{ijk} + \beta_{18} Well\_Yes_{ijk} + \beta_{19} Animal\_Yes_{ijk} \\
& + \beta_{20} Breedingsite\_Yes_{ijk} + \beta_{21} NbrNetHHS_{ijk} + \beta_{22} Season\_Rainy_{ijk}
\end{aligned}
$$

$$\beta_{0jk} = \beta_0 + v_{0k} + u_{0jk}$$

Where π_{ijk} is the predicted probability of being *P. falciparum* infection or clinical malaria positive on *i*th visit of *j*th child of the *k*th household. In this model, the level variances have to be added to the intercept. The level 2 – individual child variance, is u_{0jk} and the level 3 (household) variance is v_{0k}

The difference between conventional and the random intercept models, is the structure of the random part, also called residual variation or error. In the conventional model the structure of the residual variation is reduced to one value (visit level residual variance). In the multilevel models, the structure of the random part is more complex and partitioned among levels of the data hierarchy. The random part of the logistic model is partitioned among a visit level variance, individual level variance and household level variance. (Mauny et al 2004). The coefficients in the multilevel models were estimated using a Second Order Penalised Quasi-Likelihood (PQL) (Goldstein and Rasbash 1996). Fixed and random coefficients were successively estimated, and iterative estimations were performed until the procedure converged (Mauny et al. 2004). Statistical significance of fixed parameters and variance was tested using Wald test at 95% CI (Greenland 2000) Normal distribution of individual and household level residuals was checked graphically. STATA 8.1 was used for conventional logistic regression and MLwiN2 for multilevel modelling (Rasbash et al. 2004).

2.7.3.3 Effect of temperature rainfall and relative humidity on P. falciparum incidence The effect of mean temperature (T°C), relative humidity (RH), and rainfall (Pmm) of the previous month on *P. falciparum* infection was assessed using conventional binary response logistic regression model. As these parameters are correlated, interaction terms were included in the model. These terms were: T°C*RH, T°C*Rainfall and RH*Pmm. We also included in the model all parameters which showed a significant effect on *P. falciparum* Infection with the random effect model, described in the previous section. Since all the parameters under investigation are continuous variables and their relation with *P. falciparum* infection are not assumed to be linear, multivariate Fractional Polynomial (FP) procedures were used to examine their best fitting relationship with *P. falciparum* infection (Becher 2004, page 611). The fitting procedure involves transforming the continuous variable using a class of eight possible functions to find out the one that gives the best fit (Royston 2000). These functions are defined as follows: $H_1(X) = X^p$, where *p* takes eight possible values: -2, -1, -0.5, 0, 0.5, 1, 2, 3. The linear transformation is X^1 and X^0 is defined as the logarithm of *X*, log(*X*). The transformation can be either first-degree or second-degree.

In the first-degree, the transformation uses only one of the eight possible powers consecutively. The best fit is determined by comparing the deviances of the different models with the linear one. The model with the largest significant deviance difference from the linear one is the best fitting first-degree FP. Significance is tested using Chi-square distribution at one degree of freedom at the α=0.05. For a simple model with the one continuous variable (e.g. temperature) and one binary variable (e.g. mosquito net use, Yes/No), the logistic regression model using first degree FP will be:

$$\log it(\pi_{ib}) = \alpha + \beta_1 H_1(X_i) + \gamma W_b$$

Where π_{ib} is the predicted probability of being *P. falciparum* infection positive at temperature *i* for child using bednet *b*; γ is the coefficient of the covariable *W* use of net. H_1(X) the functional form to which the co-variable X is transformed.

The second degree transformation uses a combination of two powers from the same list of eight. In total 36, combinations are possible. This is calculated as follows:

$$C_k^n = \frac{n!}{k!(n-k)!},$$

where *n* is the number of possible powers (8), and *k* the number chosen (2), then

$$C_2^8 = \frac{8!}{2!(8-2)!} = 28 .$$

In addition, the eight combinations with the same power are added. All possible combinations are consecutively tested. The models' deviance differences from the best first-degree model are calculated and compared with the Chi-Square distribution at two degrees of freedom at α=0.05. The model with the largest significant deviance difference compared to the best *first-degree* FP is taken as the best fitting second-degree FP. Using the same example as in the first-degree FP, the second-degree FP model is mathematically defined as follows:

$$\log it(\pi_{ib}) = \alpha + \beta_1 H_1(X_i) + \beta_2 H_2(X_i) + \gamma W_b,$$

where, $H_1(X)$ and $H_2(X)$ are the respective functions through which covariate X is transformed.

All the models were run and fitted using STATA® software (StataCorp 2004).

The output (coefficients and transformed variables) of the model are then used to calculate the Rate Ratios (RR) and the predicted probability. For these models the data from Kodougou was excluded since the rainfall data was not complete.

The RR calculation was based on the reference points described in the table below.

Variables	**Reference point (x_0)**	**Rational**
Mean temperature	27°C	Value at which the risk is highest
Rainfall	164mm	Highest value observed
Relative humidity	60%	Value at which the risk is optimum

The Rate Ratio for the first-degree FP transformation is given by the function:

$$RR = \exp(\beta * (\mathrm{H}_1(X_1) - H_1(X_0)))$$

And the one for the second-degree by:

$$RR = \exp(\beta_1 * (H_1(X_1) - H_1(X_0)) + \beta_2 * (H_2(X_1) - H_2(X_0)))$$

2.7.4 Non-spatial dynamic model of malaria transmission

The dynamic concept in contrast to the static concept, tries to capture the transmission and biological processes of the disease. The model was based on the assumption the human population is divided into three categories: Susceptible (S), Malaria-infected (I) and infectious (G) and the mosquito population is classified into two compartments: non-infections (U) and infectious (Figure 2.8).

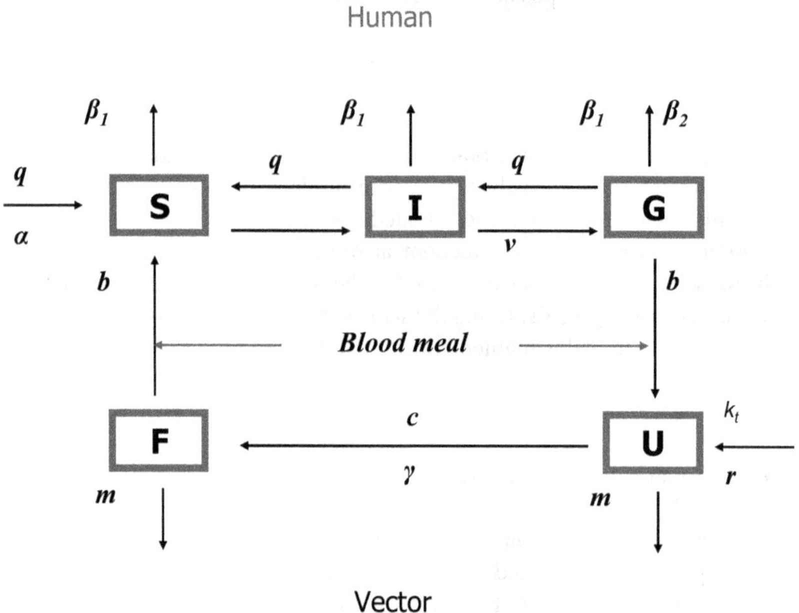

Figure 2.8 State and transition of the model

It is translated into the following five differentials equation (parameters are described in Table 2.5).

Table 2.5 Definition of model parameters

Parameters	Definition	Source
α	Natural per-capita human birth rate	DSS, in daily birth rate
β_1	Natural per-capita human death rate	DSS, in daily death rate
β_2	Malaria-induced per capita death rate in human	Noun DSS, in daily death rate
q	The malaria clearance rate in human	Fitted and compared with field data
v	Time delay for human host, from infection to infectious	Dietz et al. 1974, Gu et al. 2003
m	Daily mortality rate of vectors	From this study
r	Mosquito per-capita intrinsic growth rate	10, precise value fitted from model
B	Daily biting rate of vectors	The lower bound if 1/ gonotrophic cycle, precise value fitted from model
b	Daily rate at which a vector bites humans	b=B*HBI
γ	Probability of vector becoming infected after infectious bite	Fitted
c	Time delay for vector from infection to infectious stage	Sporogonic cycle, Detinova formula 111/(T°C-18)
K_t	Environmental carrying capacity	$K_t = Pmm*akt$

$$\delta S = \alpha(S+I+G) + q(I+G) - \left(1 - \left(\frac{S+I+G-1}{S+I+G}\right)^{bF}\right) S - \beta_1 S \tag{1}$$

$$\delta I = \left(1 - \left(\frac{S+I+G-1}{S+I+G}\right)^{bF}\right) S - (1-(\beta_1+\beta_2+q))^v \left[\left(1 - \left(\frac{S+I+G-1}{S+I+G}\right)^{bF}\right) S\right]_{t-v} - (\beta_1+\beta_2+q) I \tag{2}$$

$$\delta G = (1-(\beta_1+\beta_2+q))^v \left[\left(1 - \left(\frac{S+I+G-1}{S+I+G}\right)^{bF}\right) S\right]_{t-v} - (\beta_1+\beta_2+q) G \tag{3}$$

$$\delta U = \frac{r(U+F)}{\left[1 + \frac{(U+F)}{K_t}\right]} - \left[bU \frac{G}{S+I+G}\right]_t \gamma - mU \tag{4}$$

$$\delta F = (1-m)^c \left[bU \frac{G}{S+I+G}\right]_{t-c} \gamma - mF \tag{5}$$

Equations 1–3 describe the change in the human population while equations 4–5 describe change in vector population. Each term is explained in detail below.

2.7.4.1 Change in uninfected human population

$$\delta S = \alpha(S+I+G) + q(I+G) - \left(1 - \left(\frac{S+I+G-1}{S+I+G}\right)^{bF}\right)S - \beta_1 S \quad \textbf{(1)}$$

Equation 1 describes the changes in the uninfected human population and includes four terms:

- The first term is the natural growth rate which is expressed by $\alpha(S+I+G)$ if people born healthy and irrespective of the health of the mother. As the model is simulated daily, this is expected to be negligible.

- The second term is the malaria clearance expressed by $q(I+G)$. We assume that people clear the infection at a fixed rate from all stages of the disease. We also assume there is no immunity and no superinfection (additional infection starts after a new hepatic stage), contrary to Dietz *et al* (1974).

- The third term is the human infection expressed

$$\left(1 - \left(\frac{S+I+G-1}{S+I+G}\right)^{bF}\right)S.$$

It expresses the daily new infection within the human population.
The expression

$$\frac{S+I+G-1}{S+I+G} = 1 - \frac{1}{S+I+G}$$

is the probability of a single person not getting a bite from specific mosquito; *b*F is the number of infectious mosquito biting in a day, given a daily biting rate per mosquito of *b,*

$$\left(\frac{S+I+G-1}{S+I+G}\right)^{bF}$$

is the probability of a specific person not getting bitten by any of the infectious mosquitoes.

$$1 - \left(\frac{S+I+G-1}{S+I+G}\right)^{bF}$$

is the probability of a specific person getting bitten by one or more of infectious mosquitoes. Multiplying by S gives the number of uninfected peoples being bitten by at least one infectious mosquito in a day.

- The fourth term is $/3_l$ the death rate in the population from all causes except malaria, assuming there is not link with malaria. Then $/3_lS$ is the number of deaths within the uninfected population.

In addition the following assumptions were made:

1. A mosquito bites only once in a gonotrophic cycle.
2. Mosquitoes bite randomly. No specific attraction to any sub population.
3. The stage of infection does not influence the mosquitoes biting habits.
4. An infectious bite necessarily causes *P. falciparum* infection.

2.7.4.2 Change in infected human population

$$\delta I = \left(1-\left(\frac{S+I+G-1}{S+I+G}\right)^{bF}\right)S-(1-(\beta_1+\beta_2+q))^{v}\left[\left(1-\left(\frac{S+I+G-1}{S+I+G}\right)^{bF}\right)S\right]_{t-v}-(\beta_1+\beta_2+q)I \quad \textbf{(2)}$$

Equation 2 describes the changes in the infected (but not infectious) human population and includes three terms:

- The first term is,

  $$\left(1-\left(\frac{S+I+G-1}{S+I+G}\right)^{bF}\right)S$$

  and as described above is the number of uninfected people being bitten by at least one infectious mosquito in a day.

- The second term,

  $$\left[\left(1-\left(\frac{S+I+G-1}{S+I+G}\right)^{bF}\right)S\right]_{t-v}$$

  represents people that became infected *v* days ago. They have now mature gametocytes and are infectious. However not all of those people are still available. They may have either died of malaria of other disease or else cleared their infection. For each day the probability of leaving the group early will be $/3_l +/3_2 +q$. The probability of remaining in the group for a day is $1-(\beta_1+\beta_2+q)$. The probability of completing the whole process of *v* days is $(1-(\beta_1+\beta_2+q))^{v}$

- The third term, $-(\beta_1+\beta_2+q)I$ represents the number of people that leave the infected stage by death or clearance

In addition, the following assumptions were made:

1. /3$_2$ is constant and does not change according to the stage of the infection. We know the mortality could change per stage. We may leave it out of this equation for biological reasons.
2. q is not specific to the stage of the infection. We have two types of q. clearance due to treatment and clearance due to immune system (natural clearance). We could also decide there is no natural clearance. We also know that drugs are stage specific (liver stage, blood stage).

2.7.4.3 Change in infectious human population

$$\delta G = (1-(\beta_1+\beta_2+q))^{v}\left[\left(1-\left(\frac{S+I+G-1}{S+I+G}\right)^{bF}\right)S\right]_{t-v} - (\beta_1+\beta_2+q)G \quad \textbf{(3)}$$

Equation 3 describes the changes in the infectious human population and includes two terms.

- The first term

  $(1-(\beta_1+\beta_2+q))^{v}\left[\left(1-\left(\frac{S+I+G-1}{S+I+G}\right)^{bF}\right)S\right]_{t-v}$ is described above.

- The second term, $-(\beta_1+\beta_2+q)G$ represents the number of people that leave the infectious stage by death or clear ance

2.7.4.4 Change in the size of uninfected vector population

$$\delta U = \frac{r(U+F)}{\left[1+\frac{(U+F)}{K_t}\right]} - \left[bU\frac{G}{S+I+G}\right]_t \gamma - mU \quad \textbf{(4)}$$

Equation 4 describes the changes in the uninfected vector population and includes 3 terms.

- The first term:

  $$\frac{r(U+F)}{\left[1+\frac{(U+F)}{K_t}\right]}$$

  is the maturation of the larval stage. This term describes the number of larvae surviving to become mature mosquitoes. The numerator is the number of larvae expected to survive to maturity under ideal conditions. U+F is the total number of mosquitoes, if infectious status does not influence the fertility. r is the per mosquitoes fertility (number of eggs oviposited per day multiplied by the probability of each to develop into a mature mosquito under ideal conditions). The denominator reflects the decrease in survival because of non-ideal conditions. The *U+F* expresses the density dependent limitation on larvae survival. The precise characteristic of this dependence is determined by the carrying capacity K_t. In principle, K_t varies with temperature, rainfall and humidity and should be measured from the field. Thus the number of larvae increases with the number of mosquitoes but is limited by carrying capacity. The number of the larvae surviving is dependent on surface water available. As at this stage of research a full evapo-transpiration model is not available, K_t is therefore assumed to be proportional to the previous weekly aggregated rainfall. $K_t = Pmm*akt$. The value of *akt* is to be determined empirically.

- The second term:

$$bU\frac{G}{S+I+G},$$

is the new infections of mosquito at time *t*. *b*U is the number of uninfected mosquitoes biting in a day. The fraction is the probability of a single mosquito biting at random an infectious human out of the total human population. We multiply this by γ to reflect the probability of becoming infected.

- The third term, *mU*, is the mortality of uninfected mosquitoes, number of uninfected mosquitoes dying per day. *m* was calculated from the *k-value* (log generation mortality). In the study site setting, because of the constantly warm temperature, the gonotrophic cycle varies between 2 and 3 days. The survival of mosquitoes is per gonotrophic cycle and because of the stability of the cycle *m* was treated as constant. The precise value of *m* was empirically determined by the fit of the model.

In addition the following assumptions were made:

1. Mosquito bites randomly and independently of the infectious status
2. Survival is independent of the infectious status

2.7.4.5 Change in the size of the infectious vector population

$$\delta F = (1-m)^c \left[bU\frac{G}{S+I+G}\right]_{t-c} \gamma - mF \qquad \textbf{(5)}$$

Equation 5 describes the changes in the infected vector population and includes two terms:

- The first term:

$$(1-m)^c \left[bU \frac{G}{S+I+G} \right]_{t-c} \gamma$$

  is the number of mosquitoes infected *c* days ago, reduced by the survival. *c* is the sporogonic cycle given by Detinova (1962) as 111/(T°-18).

- The second term $-mF$ is the number of infectious mosquitoes dying in a day.

In addition the following assumptions were made:

1. Infectious mosquitoes never clear their infectious status
2. Mosquitoes are either infected or infectious

2.7.4.6 Model implementation, simulation and testing

- **Implementation of the model in Ms Excel®**
  The model was recast and implemented in Microsoft Excel® sheet in a set of difference equations with the time step of one day. This time step was chosen because it is about the biological process of the mosquito. Each of the variables (S, I, G, F and U) were followed in a separate column. In addition, at each stage the daily changes of these variables were calculated. An offset function was used for the process with delay, such as the mosquito becoming infectious at the end of the sporogonic cycle. This required a conditional test the process did not begin before the beginning of the simulation. The model is driven by temperature which defines the sporogonic cycle and by rainfall which are used in calculating the carrying capacity (k_t).

- **Optimizing and fitting the model**
  The goodness of fit was defined by the value of residual sum of square (SS) of the difference between the predicted the observed value of all months. The value of each parameter was determined successively by minimizing SS. This process was continued for all parameters until no further progress was made, which was the common minimum for all parameters. MS Excel "Solver Add-in" option function which uses the Generalized Reduced Gradient (GRG2) method was used for this process.

- **Model output and testing against observed values**
  The model was used to predict the monthly (2004) mosquito abundance and malaria incidence for each site, except Kodougou, where the rainfall

data were missing. Output values were normalised with the expected, by multiplying each predicted monthly value by a ratio. This ratio was obtained by dividing the observed highest value by the predicted value of same month.

The variance for the normalised prediction and observed values were calculated to assess the fit of the model for each site. A small variance indicates a good representation of the field data by the model. The fit was also presented graphically by plotting the monthly predicted values and the observed ones.

For the *P. falciparum* infection prediction a 95% Confidence interval was calculated for each monthly value. This was achieved by: first calculating the standard error (SE) of the two distributions, assuming a linear relationship; and then using the formula $X_i \pm 1.96 * SE$, where X is the value of a month *i*.

2.8 Ethical considerations

The study was approved by the Nouna Local Ethics committee. All participation was subject to oral informed consent.

2.8.1 Malaria survey

The children were recruited only with the consent of their parents. The study objectives and methods were explained to the parents in a digestible language. They were free to withdraw the child if they wanted to do so. All the children under study were treated, at the project cost, for malaria and other common pathologies when sick. During the weekly visit, a presumptive treatment was given to every febrile child and he/she was monitored daily for fever. The treatment was done according to the national guidelines for malaria chemotherapy (CQ: 25 mg/kg weight during three days; day one and two: 10 mg/kg, single intake; day three: 5 mg/kg). In case of no improvement, the child was referred to the nearest health centre, and the district referral hospital. All medical and related costs were covered by the project. A basic training on malaria treatment and recognition of dangers signs was given to the interviewers.

Single use lancets were used for finger pricks in each child. The method caused a slight discomfort, but no risk of being infected by other pathogens. A strong safety procedure was applied to protect the children and the interviewers from contamination. Although the name, sex and age of the participant were recorded in the survey, the identity of the participants was not associated with any publication.

2.8.2 Entomological survey

2.8.2.1 Light trap capture Houses were used on the agreement of the head of household. People inside the house were protected with mosquito net, and that insured minimum risk to the residents.

2.8.2.2 Human land capture Since this was the most risky method, capturers were recruited upon informed consent. They were given malaria prophylaxis and monitored for fever and parasite infection for two weeks after captures took place. All sick capturers were treated at the project's cost. In addition, they received a token financial incentive.

2.8.2.3 Pyrethrum spray capture Inhabitants were asked to leave the house before the spray of the insecticide. Food, water or any container in the house was carefully covered to avoid any possible contamination. Occupants were able to re-enter the house 15 minutes after the spray. Low dosage of the insecticide was applied and spraying lasted for less that three minutes.

2.8.3 Weather monitoring

Not risky for human subjects. However, consent was obtained from the village chief before installation of the meteorological stations.

Chapter 3
Results

3.1 Characteristics of the study population

Table 3.1 gives a summary of the population characteristics at the beginning of the study. In total, 867 children took part in the study. They were from Cissé (171), Goni (240), Koudougou (191) and Nouna (265). Participants were distributed in 427 households giving an overall mean of 2.0 under five children per household. The highest number of children per household was observed in Kodougou (2.5) and the lowest in Nouna (1.8). The sex distribution was not significantly different across the sites (Chi square test, p=0.421). Overall, females (52.5%) were more than males. The age distribution across the sites was not significantly different (Chi square test, p=0.562) although, children were slightly younger in Nouna, with a mean age of 31.7 months (standard deviation: 15.0) compared to Cissé (mean age 34.7 months). Overall, except the age group below 12 months (9.2%), participants were almost equally distributed in the age groups 12–23 months (23.1%), 24–35 months (23.4%), 36–47 (24.3%) and older than 48 months (20.1%). This pattern was consistent in all sites, except Kodougou, where a slightly higher proportion was observed in the age group 36–47 months (26.2%). The ethnic distribution was significantly different between sites (Chi square test, p>0.0001). Overall the majority were Marka and Mossi representing respectively 31.4% and 30.3% of the study population. Bwaba were the minority (7.5%). In Cissé 84.2% of the participants were Fulani. Marka ethnic group was the majority in Goni (68.8%) and Nouna (33.3%). Children from Kodougou were predominantly Mossi (72.8%). Nouna had the particularity that, differences between the ethnic group proportions were not high as compared to the other sites (Table 3.1).

At the end of the study, 839 children remained. The distribution according to the household, sex, age group and ethnic group is given in Table 3.2. As expected, they were no children any more in the age group below 12 months and 20.4% grew over 59 months. The age distribution across sites was significantly different (Chi square test p=0.025). In Cissé the highest proportion belonged to the age group 60+ (25.9), in Goni it was 36–47 months (25.4%), Kodougou 48–59 months (26.8%) and Nouna, equally 36–47 months (24.0%) and 48–59 months (24%). The mean age remained higher in Cissé (46.3 month, standard deviation of 15.4). The sex and ethnic distribution remained similar to the one at the beginning of the follow-up.

Table 3.1 Characteristics of the study population at the beginning of the study (01.12.03)

	All	(%)	Site								
			Cissé	(%)	Goni	(%)	Kod*	(%)	Nouna	(%)	** x^2 test
n	867		171		240		191		265		-
Household	427	-	74	-	125	-	77	-	151	-	-
Children/HH	2.0	-	2.3	-	1.9	-	2.5	-	1.8	-	-
Gender											*P=0.421*
Female	455	(52.5)	103	(60.2)	116	(48.3)	98	(51.3)	138	(52.1)	
Male	412	(47.5)	68	(39.8)	124	(51.7)	93	(48.7)	127	(47.9)	
Age (Month)											*p=0.562*
<12	80	(9.2)	14	(8.2)	19	(7.9)	15	(7.9)	32	(12.1)	
12–23	200	(23.1)	39	(22.8)	57	(23.8)	43	(22.5)	61	(23)	
24–35	202	(23.3)	36	(21.1)	59	(24.6)	43	(22.5)	64	(24.2)	
36–47	211	(24.3)	40	(23.4)	58	(24.2)	50	(26.2)	63	(23.8)	
48–59	174	(20.1)	42	(24.6)	47	(19.6)	40	(20.9)	45	(17)	
Ethnic											*p=0.001*
Bwaba	65	(7.5)	2	(1.2)	4	(1.7)	32	(16.8)	27	(10.2)	
Fulany	171	(19.7)	144	(84.2)	5	(2.1)	-	-	22	(8.3)	
Marka	272	(31.4)	18	(10.5)	165	(68.8)	1	(0.5)	88	(33.2)	
Mossi	263	(30.3)	1	(0.6)	66	(27.5)	139	(72.8)	57	(21.5)	
Samo	83	(9.6)	4	(2.3)	0	(0)	17	(8.9)	62	(23.4)	
Others	13	(1.5)	2	(1.2)	0	(0)	2	(1)	9	(3.4)	

* Kodougou, ** Mantel-Haenszel chi-Square, test for difference across sites. P-value<0.0= significant difference

Table 3.2 Characteristics of the study population at the end of the study (30.12.04)

	Sites										
	All	**(%)**	**Cissé**	**(%)**	**Goni**	**(%)**	**Kod***	**(%)**	**Nouna**	**(%)**	*****x² test***
	839		**162**		**232**		**183**		**262**		-
Household	422	-	74		122		76		150		-
Children/HH	2.0	-	2.2		1.9		2.4		1.7		-
Gender											p=0.455
Female	437	52.1	100	(61.7)	109	(47)	91	(49.7)	137	(52.3)	
Male	402	47.9	62	(38.3)	123	(53)	92	(50.3)	125	(47.7)	
Age (Month											p=0.025
<12	0	0.0	0	(0)	0	(0)	0	(0)	0	(0)	
12-23	71	8.5	12	(7.4)	16	(6.9)	11	(6)	32	(12.2)	
24-35	193	23.0	36	(22.2)	56	(24.1)	42	(23)	59	(22.5)	
36-47	198	23.6	34	(21)	59	(25.4)	42	(23)	63	(24)	
48-59	206	24.6	38	(23.5)	56	(24.1)	49	(26.8)	63	(24)	
60+	171	20.4	42	(25.9)	45	(19.4)	39	(21.3)	45	(17.2)	
Mean Age(SD)	44.5(15.1)		46.3 (15.4)		44.4 (15.0)		45.5 (14.9)		42.8(15.0)		
Ethnic											p<0.0001
Bwaba	64	7.6	2	(1.2)	4	(1.7)	31	(16.9)	27	(10.3)	
Fulany	162	19.3	135	(83.3)	5	(2.2)	0	(0)	22	(8.4)	
Marka	263	31.3	18	(11.1)	157	(67.7)	0	(0)	88	(33.6)	
Mossi	255	30.4	1	(0.6)	66	(28.4)	133	(72.7)	55	(21)	
Samo	82	9.8	4	(2.5)	0	(0)	17	(9.3)	61	(23.3)	
Others	13	1.5	2	(1.2)	0	(0)	2	(1.1)	9	(3.4)	

* Kodougou, ** Mantel-Haenszel chi-Square, test for difference across sites. P-value<0.0= significant difference

3.2 Outcome of follow up

Follow up started on 01.12.2003. 52 home visits per child were planned, but on average each child was observed for 45.43 weeks. During follow up, 38 children (4.4% of 867) left the cohort because of death (15) and migration out of the study sites (13) The number of dropouts was less in Nouna (3 children) compared to the other three sites (Cissé=9, Goni=8 and Kodougou=4) (Figure 3.1). Children were not always present at each visit therefore the person time observed is different from the number of children (Figure 3.1). Overall 109.0 (867–758.0) person-years (PY) were lost, with a difference between sites. The highest number was observed in Nouna (45.8 PY) followed by Kodougou (27.9 PY), Cissé (20 PY) and Goni (15.6 PY).

Over the observation time the weekly response rate (children present at the visit) varied. In Figure 3.2, the weekly response is plotted for each site and for

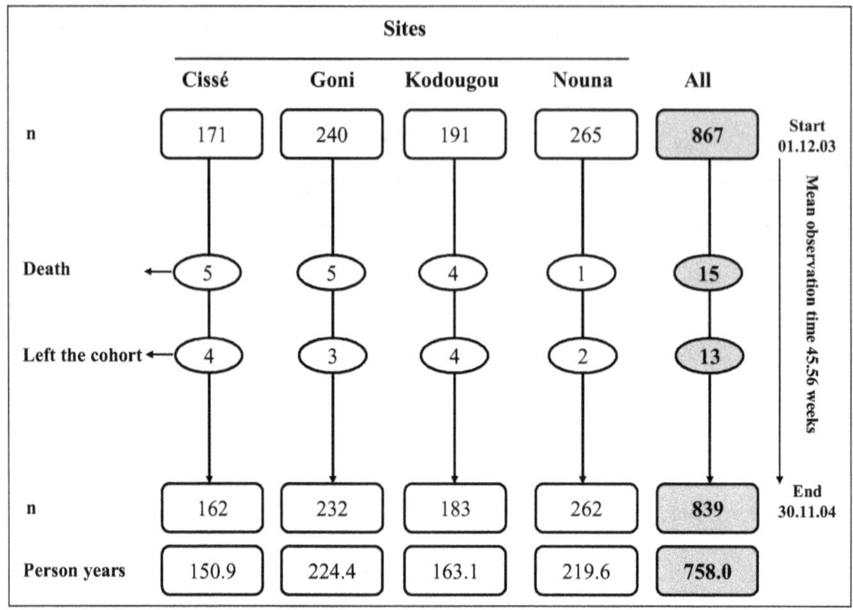

Figure 3.1 Follow-up status of the study participants

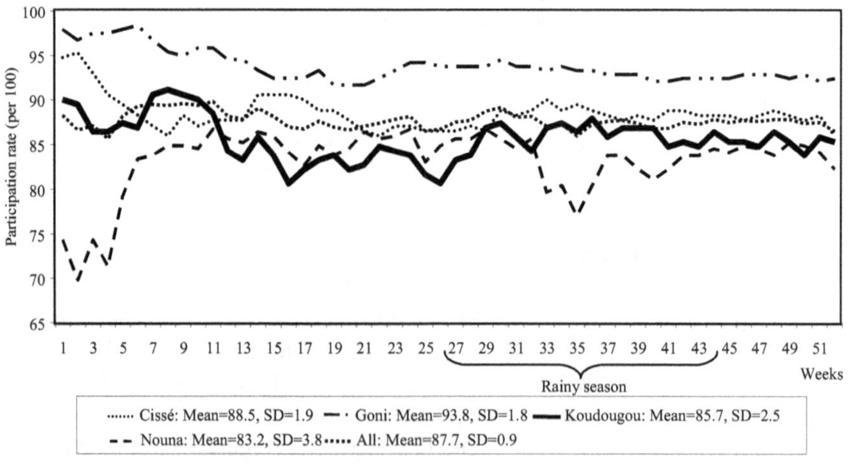

Figure 3.2 Weekly response rate per site

all sites combined. We observed the response rate was not constant overtime for all sites. The overall mean participation rate over the observation period was 87.7% with a small variation (Standard Deviation (SD) of 0.9). In Nouna, it was particularly low with a large variation (mean =83.2%, SD=3.8), where we observed low rates from the week 1 to 5 and from 32 to 35. Goni had the highest participation rate (93.8%, SD=1.8) with small variation over time. In Cissé, the participation rate was higher (above 90%) in the first weeks (1 to 3), but dropped and remained around 89%. In Kodougou where the second lowest mean rate was observed (85.7%) the variation overtime was high (SD=2.46). The lowest rates were observed from the visit number 15 to 27.

3.3 Fever and *P. falciparum* infection status

A summary of fever *P. falciparum* infection status in the study participants is given in Figure 3.3. Overall 1635 episodes of fever (armpit temperature >=37.5°C) were observed. This gives an incidence of 2.2 episodes per person year (1635 episodes /758.0 person years) during the observation period. The incidence of fever episodes per person year was similar in all sites (Cissé= 2.1, Goni=2.3, Kodougou=2.2 and Nouna=2.0). Among 1635 fever episodes 844 tested positive for *P. falciparum* infection, giving a *P. falciparum* crude infection incidences of 1.1 episodes per person year. The lowest incidence was observed in Nouna where children got less that 1 episode (0.8). In Cissé, Goni and Kodougou the incidence were 1.2, 1.3, 1.4, respectively. Out of 844 episodes tested *P. falciparum* infection positive 597 presented a parasite load of =>5,000 parasite/μl, fulfilling the definition of clinical malaria. The number of malaria episodes per person year, was higher in Kodougou (1.0) and lower in Nouna (0.5). It was 0.8 and 0.9 respectively in Cissé and Goni. Severe malaria episodes incidence, defined as fever plus parasite load of >=100,000/μl were low in all sites (Cissé= 0.1, Goni=0.1, Kodougou=0.1 and Nouna=0.2)

3.3.1 Monthly P. falciparum infection incidence

We observed a strong monthly variation of *P. falciparum* infection incidence among the study population. The lowest incidence rates per 1,000 person years were consistently observed for all sites in May and June (Cissé: 6.7, 6.3; Goni: 31.0, 29.1; Kodougou: 18.5, 17.6 and Nouna: 22.0, 12.4) (Table 3.3). The overall incidences were respectively 25.4 and 21.0 per 1,000. In contrast, the highest incidence was observed in different months for each site. It was in September for Goni (272.6 per 1,000 person years), December 2003 for Kodougou (239.1 per 1,000 person years), August for Cissé (268.6 per 1,000 person years) and October for Nouna (126.5 per 1,000 person years) (Table 3.3).

Figure 3.4 shows *P. falciparum* infection incidence rate per 1,000 person years plotted for each site and per month. As the difference between the smallest and

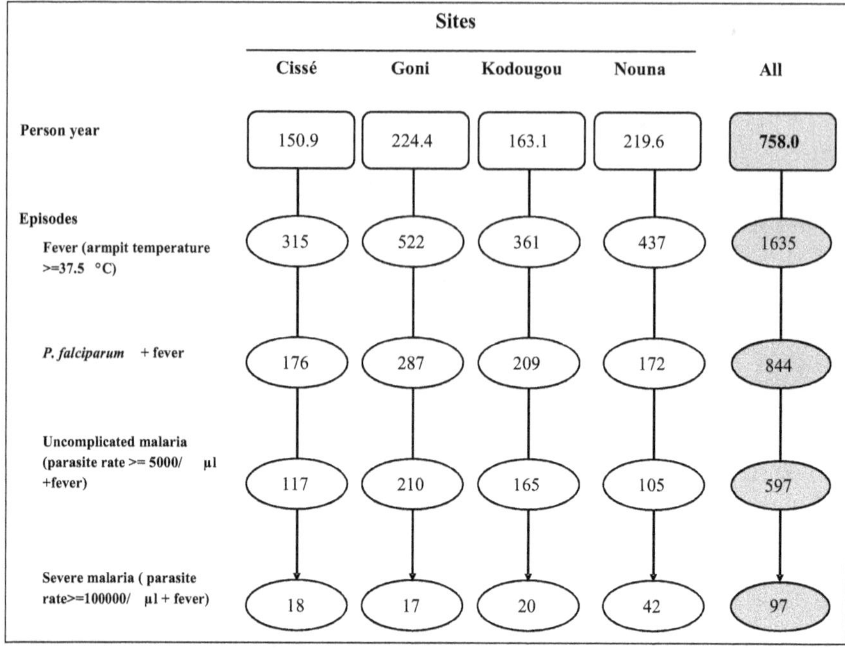

Figure 3.3 *P. falciparum* infection status among participants at the end of the follow-up

Table 3.3 Distribution of *P. falciparum* infection incidence per month and sites among study children

	Cissé			Goni			Kodougou			Nouna			All		
Month	PM	C	IR (1000)	PM	C	IR (1000)	PM	C	IR (1000)	PM	C	IR (1000)	PM	C	IR (1000)
Dec 03	149.8	29	159.2	221.4	27	122.0	158.9	38	239.1	185.0	20	88.9	715.1	114	159.4
Jan-04	139.5	6	43.6	215.8	8	37.6	160.1	12	76.1	208.4	7	34.1	723.8	33	45.6
Feb-04	139.8	19	137.9	213.3	8	38.1	154.2	10	65.4	211.6	12	57.5	718.9	49	68.2
Mar 04	145.9	18	123.4	210.8	18	85.4	150.2	11	60.2	212.6	11	42.6	719.5	58	80.6
Apr-04	139.3	2	14.6	205.8	12	59.2	148.6	3	20.5	210.5	26	125.3	704.2	43	61.1
May 04	123.2	1	6.7	185.6	7	31.0	133.6	3	18.5	187.3	5	22.0	629.6	16	25.4
Jun-04	130.7	1	6.3	198.1	7	29.1	140.2	3	17.6	198.3	3	12.4	667.3	14	21.0
Jul-04	142.6	2	14.2	209.5	23	111.4	153.8	12	79.2	199.5	7	35.6	705.4	44	62.4
Aug-04	131.7	43	268.6	197.5	53	220.7	148.5	32	177.3	197.7	20	83.2	675.4	148	219.1
Sep-04	125.6	25	163.7	181.1	60	272.6	131.9	37	230.8	176.1	23	107.0	614.7	145	235.9
Oct 04	140.9	18	129.6	207.9	41	200.1	152.4	28	186.4	208.6	26	126.5	709.8	113	159.2
Nov-04	139.8	12	87.1	207.2	23	112.6	151.7	20	133.8	208.1	12	58.5	706.8	67	94.8
Total	**150.9**	**176**	**1166.4**	**224.4**	**287**	**1278.7**	**163.1**	**209**	**1281.6**	**219.6**	**152**	**692.1**	**758.0**	**844**	**1113.4**

PM: Person month, C: cases, IR (1,000): Incidence rate per 1,000

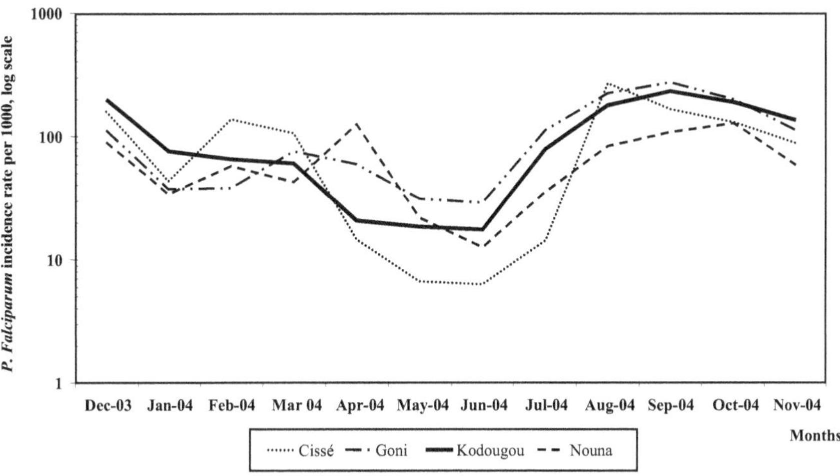

Figure 3.4 ***P. falciparum* infection incidence rate, per month and site**

the highest rate was large (272.6–6.3=266.6), the rates are shown on a logarithmic scale. For all sites the incidence rate decreased from December to June where it reached the lowest level. It started rising again in July to reach a peak in August, September and October then dropped. Cissé curve shows a different pattern compared to the other sites. The incidence dropped from December 2003 to January 2004 then rose in February and remained high in March before dropping again in April. While in the three other sites a decrease of the incidence rate was observed in April, in Nouna there was a peak.

3.3.2 Monthly clinical malaria

Clinical malaria incidence followed the same pattern as the *P. falciparum* infection. Table 3.4 shows an overall incidence per 1,000 person years of 520 episodes/758.0 person years. Over the study period the incidence was less than one episode per child. This incidence rate varies according to the site with Goni having the highest (834.0 episodes per 1,000 person years) and Nouna the lowest (409.8 per 1,000 person years). The monthly incidence varies consistently across sites. The highest incidence was observed in August, September and October and November. Figure 3.5 shows a decrease of the incidence from December 2003 to January 2004, which then remained low until June where it rises to reach a peak in September for Goni and Kodougou (287.2 and 265.4 per 1,000 person years, respectively). For Cissé, the incidence rose a month later in July and reach a peak earlier in august (303.8 per ,000 person years). In Nouna, the peak was observed in October (79.5 per 1,000 person year), however the highest incidence was in December 2003 (81.1 per 1,000 person years).

Table 3.4 Distribution of clinical malaria incidence per month and sites among study children

Month	Cissé			Goni			Kodougou			Nouna			All		
	PM	C	IR (1000)	PM	C	IR (1000)	PM	C	IR (1000)	PM	C	IR (1000)	PM	C	IR (1000)
Dec 03	149.8	16	106.8	221.4	18	81.3	158.9	29	182.5	185.0	15	81.1	715.1	78	109.1
Jan-04	139.5	5	35.8	215.8	7	32.4	160.1	5	31.2	208.4	3	14.4	723.8	20	27.6
Feb-04	139.8	7	50.1	213.3	6	28.1	154.2	7	45.4	211.6	3	14.2	718.9	23	32.0
Mar 04	145.9	7	48.0	210.8	6	28.5	150.2	7	46.6	212.6	6	28.2	719.5	26	36.1
Apr-04	139.3	0	0.0	205.8	2	9.7	148.6	2	13.5	210.5	16	76.0	704.2	20	28.4
May 04	123.2	1	8.1	185.6	1	5.4	133.6	2	15.0	187.3	3	16.0	629.6	7	11.1
Jun-04	130.7	0	0.0	198.1	3	15.1	140.2	3	21.4	198.3	2	10.1	667.3	8	12.0
Jul-04	142.6	1	7.0	209.5	18	85.9	153.8	10	65.0	199.5	6	30.1	705.4	35	49.6
Aug-04	131.7	40	303.8	197.5	42	212.6	148.5	26	175.1	197.7	13	65.8	675.4	121	179.2
Sep-04	125.6	20	159.2	181.1	52	287.2	131.9	35	265.4	176.1	14	79.5	614.7	121	196.9
Oct 04	140.9	15	106.4	207.9	34	163.5	152.4	23	151.0	208.6	15	71.9	709.8	87	122.6
Nov-04	139.8	6	42.9	207.2	21	101.4	151.7	16	105.5	208.1	9	43.2	706.8	52	73.6
Total	**150.9**	**102**	**676.0**	**224.4**	**192**	**855.5**	**163.1**	**136**	**834.0**	**219.6**	**90**	**409.8**	**758.0**	**520**	**686.0**

PM: Person month, C: cases, IR (1,000): Incidence rate per 1,000, Clinical malaria =fever + parasite density =>5,000µ/l

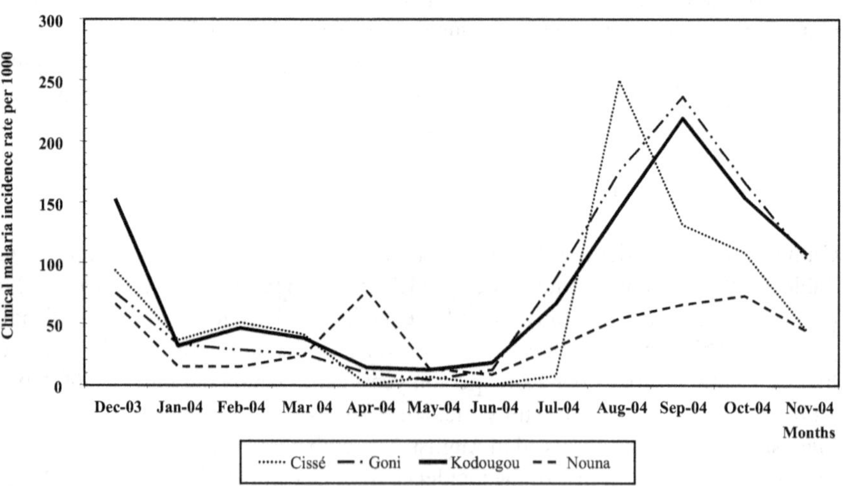

Figure 3.5 Monthly incidence rate of clinical malaria

Parasite density shows a clear age pattern and very wide variation between children within the same age group. At a young age the density is very low (below 12 months, mean=7,636.8, SD=7,033.0). The mean trophozoite density in Kodougou was highest (39,322.5μ/l) with a high standard deviation (62,229.1 μ/l) compared to the other sites which were similar (Cissé=33,535.9 μ/l, Goni=32,888.3 μ/l and Nouna=33,441.67 μ/l). Children within the age group 24–35 months had the highest parasite density (mean=38,489.5 μ/l, SD=65848.1). Older children (age group 48 months plus) had the lowest parastie density with a mean=33,357.5μ/l and SD=50,149.5) (Table 3.5).

Table 3.5 *P. falciparum* density among infected children

	Episodes	Mean	Min	Max	SD
Site					
Cissé	176	33,535.9	50	300,000	5,5162.3
Goni	287	32,888.3	50	400,000	5,5761.8
Kodougou	209	39,322.5	100	500,000	6,2296.1
Nouna	172	33,441.7	200	370,000	5,6626.0
Age					
<12	19	7,636.8	200	20,000	7,034.0
12–23	204	31,957.4	200	500,000	58,139.3
24–35	219	38,489.5	100	400,000	65,848.1
36–47	196	37,481.5	100	430,000	56,152.8
>48	206	33,357.5	50	280,000	50,49.5

3.3.3 Effect of site of residence on P. falciparum infection

P. falciparum infection incidence within a site did not show a clear spatial pattern. However, infection was clustered in some households.

The results of the multivariate conventional and random effects logistic regression models assessing the effect of site (as an ecological setting) on *P. falciparum* infection odds are presented in Table 3.6. Also included are the person years and the number of observed cases per covariable.

The results of the conventional model (model A) indicate the odds of *P. falciparum* infection for children living in Cissé were similar to those from Nouna. The OR was 1.0 (95%CI: 0.7; 1.4). In Goni, the odds compared to Nouna increased by 0.20 indicating a relatively higher risk of *P. falciparum* infection of borderline significance. Children in Kodougou have a significantly higher risk (OR 1.7 95%CI: 1.4; 2.0) of getting infected by *P. falciparum*. Among other covariates, only age, treatment, "presence of farm" and "rainy season" showed a significant effect. When the children were classified into five age group of 12 months interval and the oldest group was taken as reference category, we observed the odds of *P. falciparum* infection decreased significantly with increasing age. The odds of infection were 2.6 times in children below 12 months and 1.4 for those between 36–47 months. The covariable "Treated at previous visit" indicates children who had fever at the preceding visit and were given Chloroquine. The model (A) shows an OR of 0.3 (95%CI: 0.3; 0.9), suggesting a significant reduction of odds for treated children. Farming within 30-metre radius of the household was significantly associated with an increase of the odds of *P. falciparum* infection. Other housing condition factors such as house type, presence of well, presence of animal and breeding sites did not show any effect. *P. falciparum* infection among children showed a seasonal effect. The rainy season was defined as a period between the June and October. The rainy season was associated with significantly increased risk of infection. The OR in the rainy season compared to dry season was 1.6 (95%CI: 1.5; 1.8).

After accounting for the random effects at the individual and household level and assuming non-independence of the subjects, the effect of the site on *P. falciparum* infection risk was cancelled (OR Kodougou 1.1 95%CI: 0.9;1.4) (Model B). The odds of *P. falciparum* infection, after controlling for all possible confounders are therefore similar across sites. The variance estimates were significant for both levels (individual level 0.121, standard error 0.072 and household level: 0.052, standard error 0.048). Except for the effects of mosquito net use and age, all the effects of other covariates remained the same. The effect of mosquito net use changed from non-significant (Model A; OR: 1.1, 96%CI: 0.0; 1.3) to significant (Model B; OR: 1.4, 96%CI: 1.2; 1.5). In contrast to mosquito net use, the age effect changed from significant to non-significant. For example in model A, the OR for age group below 12 which was 2.6 (95%CI: 2.1; 3.1) became 0.9 (95%CI: 0.4; 1.4).

3.4 Weather variation in the four sites

As mentioned earlier, the weather station for the site of Goni was located in Toni. Rainfall data for Kodougou was partly missing and will therefore not be considered in describing the results.

Weather showed a similar pattern in all the four sites. Figure 3.6 shows a plot of weekly average temperature (°C), relative humidity (%) and total rainfall (Pmm). Rainfall was observed in all sites in the weeks 17 to 45, with a peak in the 35th week. This period corresponds to the July to October period. The total amount of rainfall observed was higher in Nouna (508. 3 mm in 68 days) compared to Cissé (334 mm in 49 days) and Toni/Goni (408.5 mm in 54 days). The relative humidity pattern followed the rainfall pattern. In all sites, it was low in first 13 weeks, and then increased from the 13th week to reach a peak in the 35th week after which

Table 3.6 Conventional and random effects logistic regression models of the effects of "site" on the odds of *P. falciparum* infection

					Model A	Model B
		Categories	**PY**	**Cases**	**OR(95% CI)**	**OR (95% CI)**
All			758.0	844		
	Variables					
	Site (explanatory)	Nouna	219.6	172	1	1
		Cissé	150.9	176	1 (0.7 – 1.4)	1 (0.7 – 1.3)
		Goni	224.4	287	**1.2 (1 – 1.5)**	1 (0.8 – 1.2)
		Kodougou	163.1	209	**1.7 (1.4 – 2)**	1.1 (0.9 – 1.4)
Individual level						
	Gender	Female	390.4	448	1	1
		Male	367.6	396	1 (0.9 – 1.1)	1 (0.9 – 1.2)
	Age in month	<=12	14.7	21	**2.6 (2.1 – 3.1)**	0.9 (0.4 – 1.4)
		12–23	149.3	214	**2 (1.8 – 2.2)**	0.8 (0.6 – 1)
		24–36	168.4	218	**1.7 (1.5 – 1.9)**	0.9 (0.7 – 1.1)
		36–47	178.7	192	**1.4 (1.2 – 1.6)**	0.8 (0.6 – 1)
		48+	246.8	199	1	1
	Ethnic	Peulh	151.5	175	1	1
		Mossi	219.2	234	0.7 (0.4 – 1)	0.9 (0.5 – 1.2)
		Marka	247.7	306	1.1 (0.8 – 1.4)	0.8 (0.5 – 1.2)
		Bwaba	59.6	69	0.9 (0.5 – 1.3)	0.9 (0.5 – 1.3)
		Samo	69.3	53	0.7 (0.3 – 1.1)	0.9 (0.5 – 1.3)
		Others	10.7	7	0.8 (0 – 1.6)	1.1 (0.5 – 1.7)
	Net use	Yes	301.7	406	1.1 (0.9 – 1.3)	**1.4 (1.2 – 1.5)**
	Treatment previous visit	Yes	23.5	11	**0.3 (-0.3 – 0.9)**	**0.3 (-0.3 – 0.9)**
Household level						
	Wall	Mud block	727	834	1	1
		Concret	31	10	0.4 (-0.3 – 1)	0.3 (-0.4 – 1)
	Roof	Iron sheet	158.4	132	1	1
		Mud	552.2	652	1.1 (0.9 – 1.3)	0.9 (0.7 – 1.1)
		Grass	47.4	60	1.1 (0.7 – 1.4)	1 (0.6 – 1.3)
	Presence of well	Yes	104.3	106	1 (0.7 – 1.3)	0.9 (0.6 – 1.2)
	Presence of farm	Yes	281.3	434	**1.5 (1.3 – 1.6)**	**1.5 (1.4 – 1.7)**
	Presence of animal	Yes	491.1	537	1 (0.8 – 1.2)	0.9 (0.7 – 1.1)
	Presence of breeding site	Yes	60.7	65	0.9 (0.5 – 1.2)	0.9 (0.6 – 1.3)
	Ratio net size of household	<1	752.0	838	1	1
		>1	6.0	6	1.2 (0.4 – 2)	1.3 (0.3 – 2.2)
	Rain season	Yes	314.5	464	**1.6 (1.5 – 1.8)**	**1.5 (1.3 – 1.6)**
	Random part					
	Household level variance					**0.052 (0.048)**
	Individual level variance					**0.121 (0.072)**

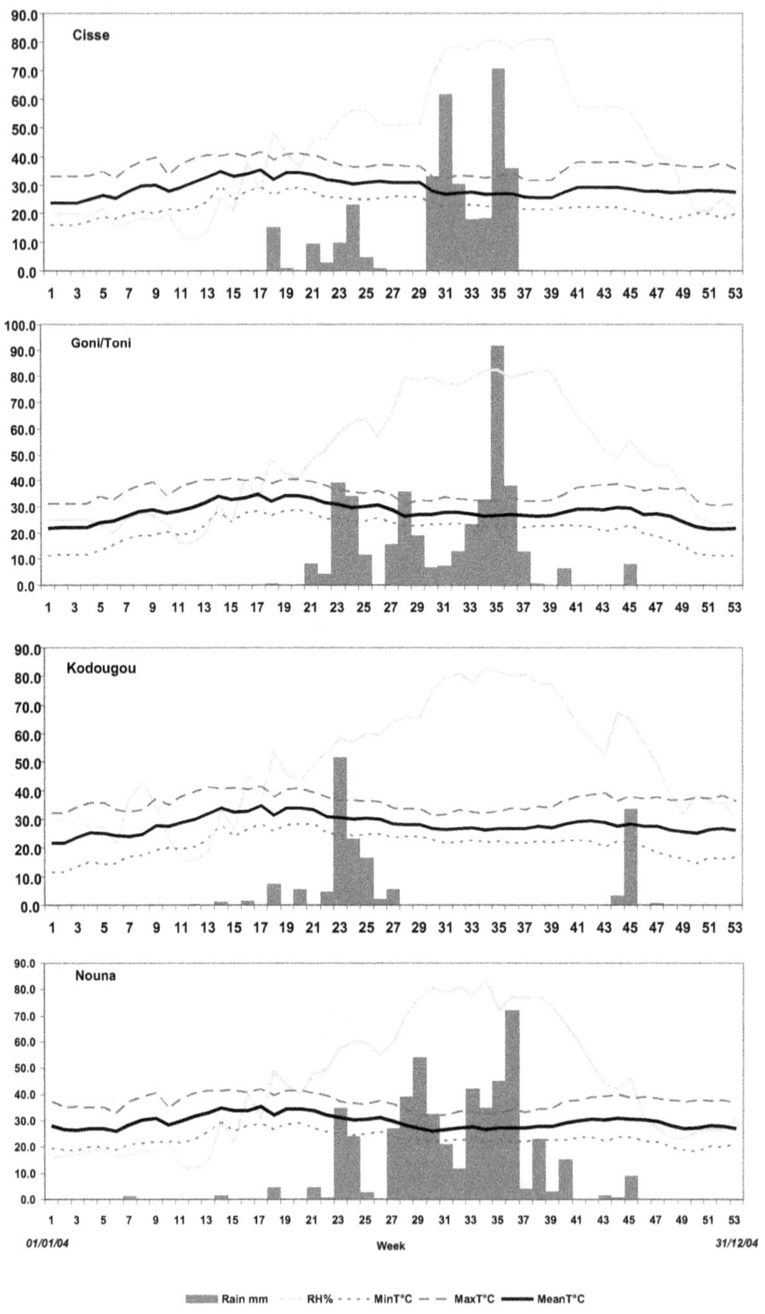

Figure 3.6 **Weekly rainfall, relative humidity and temperature (Rainfall data for Kodougou station were missing from week 28 to 48 because of sensor failure)**

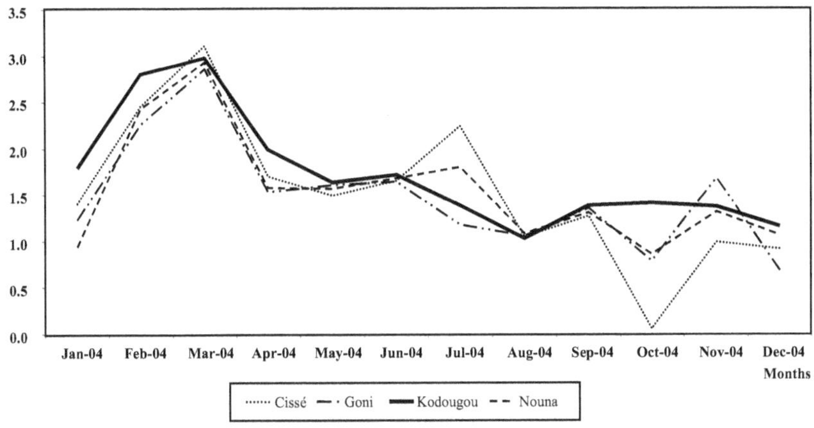

Figure 3.7 Standard deviation of daily mean temperature in each month

it decreased progressively. The average relative humidity was relatively higher in Kodougou (50.3%, range 11.3–93.3, SD: 20.7) and Toni/Goni (48.5% range 10.2–89.8, SD: 22.8) compared to Cissé (43.7%, range: 9.5-89.6, SD: 23.1) and Nouna (44.0% range: 10.4–89.4, SD: 23.8). The temperature was more or less similar in all the sites. Mean, maxima and minima temperature increased from week one to week 17 (April) where the peak was observed. At this point the mean temperature was 35.2°C (Cissé), 34.8°C (Toni/Goni), 34.6°C (Kodougou) and 35.4°C for Nouna. With the onset of the rains, the temperature decreased up to 26.6°C (for Cissé and Nouna), 26.5°C (Toni/Goni), 26.5 (Kodougou) between weeks 35 and 38 (in August and September). From then on, temperatures rose again and remained more or less constant in October-November, until they started decreasing in December, the coldest month. The average mean temperature was lower in Toni/Goni, however with high variation (27.9°C, range: 20.8–35.9, SD: 3.8) compared to Cissé (29.1°C range 22.8–35.9, SD: 3.1), Kodougou, (28.2°C range 20.8–35.9, SD 3.3) and Nouna (29.6 °C range 20.6–35.4, SD 2.9).

Daily mean temperature variation in a month expressed by the standard deviation was high in March for all sites (Cissé: 3.1, Toni/Goni: 2.9, Kodougou: 3.0, and Nouna: 2.9) as seen in Figure 3.7. From March, in all sites, this variation decreased to reach the smallest value in December for Toni/Goni: 0.7, Kodougou: 1.2, and Nouna: 1.1 An unusually small variation was observed in Cissé in October (0.1).

3.5 Effect of weather on *P. falciparum* infection

Using logistic regression with the fractional polynomial approach, we estimated the effect of weather parameter values from the previous month, on *P. falciparum* infection. The transformation functions for each variable are presented in Table 3.7. The relationships between weather parameters and *P. falciparum* infection were not linear as observed in the table. Only the combinations temperature-humidity (TRH) and temperature-rainfall (TPmm) showed linear relationships. The best fit of the models for mean temperature (Tmean), rainfall (Pmm) and relative humidity (RH) alone were obtained after second-degree transformations. The powers and transformation functions for each of the covariates are given in Table 3.7. For the combination rainfall and humidity the first-degree of transformation with a power of -1 yielded the best fit.

Table 3.7 Transformation functions of different covariates used in logistic regression models

Variable (Degree)	Variable (power)	Transformation functions
Mean temperature (1st degree)	Tmean_1 (-2)	$\left(\frac{Tmean}{10}\right)^{-2} - 0.1201$
	Tmean_2 (0.5)	$\left(\frac{Tmean}{10}\right)^{0.5} - 0.1699$
Rainfall (2nd degree)	Pmm_1 (2)	$\left(\frac{Pmm + 0.3000}{100}\right)^{2} - 0.1261$
	Pmm_2 (2)	$\left(\frac{Pmm + 0.3000}{100}\right)^{2} * \ln\left(\frac{Pmm + 0.3000}{100}\right) + 0.1306$
Relative humidity (2nd degree)	RH_1 (-1)	$\left(\frac{RH}{10}\right)^{-1} - 0.2201$
	RH_2 (-1)	$\left(\frac{RH}{10}\right)^{-1} * \ln\left(\frac{RH}{10}\right) - 0.3332$
Rainfall and humidity (1st degree)	PmmRH (-1)	$\left(\frac{PmmRH + 2.46999741}{10000}\right)^{-1} - 3.971$
Temperature and humidity (1st degree)	TRH (1)	$TRH - 1305$
Temperature and rainfall (1stdegree)	TPmm (1)	$TPmm - 989.7$

Although other covariates were included in the model for adjustment purposes, their estimates are not shown in Table 3.7 because the focus is on the weather parameters. For each power of transformation the estimate is given. The constants included in the transformation functions are for purposes of stabilising the estimates. The estimates for each variable are given in Table 3.8. All variables individually or combined had a significant effect on *P. falciparum* infection. The highest effect was observed with mean temperature. The combined effect of rainfall-humidity, temperature-humidity and temperature-rainfall, though significant was small.

Table 3.8 Model estimates and confidence limits

Variables	β estimate	95% Confidence Limit
Tmean_1	-86.9789	(-113.4057 ; -60.5521)
Tmean_2	-29.7873	(-38.7457 ; -20.8288)
Pmm_1	3.7666	(1.5279 ; 6.0053)
Pmm_2	-3.4380	(-5.3612 ; -1.5147)
RH_1	-8.9203	(-14.807 ; -3.0337)
RH_2	-23.2151	(-36.7151 ; -9.7152)
PmmRH	-0.0003	(-0.0004 ; -0.0002)
TRH	-0.0035	(-0.0058 ; -0.0012)
TPmm	-0.0012	(-0.0021 ; -0.0004)
Intercept	-3.8180	(-4.18581 ; -3.4502)

Log pseudo-likelihood=-2920.2374, Wald chi square=282, Deviance: 5840.466

The direction of the weather parameter effect on *P. falciparum* infection cannot be only defined by the β estimates, since the relationships are non linear. To better perceive the effect we have calculated the rate ratios, RR (calculation procedure describe in methods section) and plotted them (Figure 3.8). The Y axis represents the RR and the X axis the different parameters. For each parameter the reference point is indicated by vertical and horizontal lines. As the effects of the combined variables were not strong, their RR were not calculated.

For mean temperature the reference point used was 27°C. Temperatures observed ranged from 21°C to 34°C. The relationship of mean temperature and *P. falciparum* infection showed a “bell shape” pattern (Figure 3.8a). The risk of *P. falciparum* infection increased with the increase of mean temperature up to 27°C. At 23°C there was a risk reduction of 53% compared to 27°C. Temperatures above 27°C led to a significant decrease of *P. falciparum* infection risk. The risk was minimal at lower and higher mean temperature.

The RR for rainfall was calculated using 164 mm as a reference point. This point corresponds to the maximum rainfall value observed. The effect of rainfall on *P. falciparum* infection risk was only observed for values above 100mm (Figure 3.8b). Below that level the risk reduction compared to 164 mm was almost 100%. There was no difference in effect for rainfall values of 60mm or 90 mm. Above

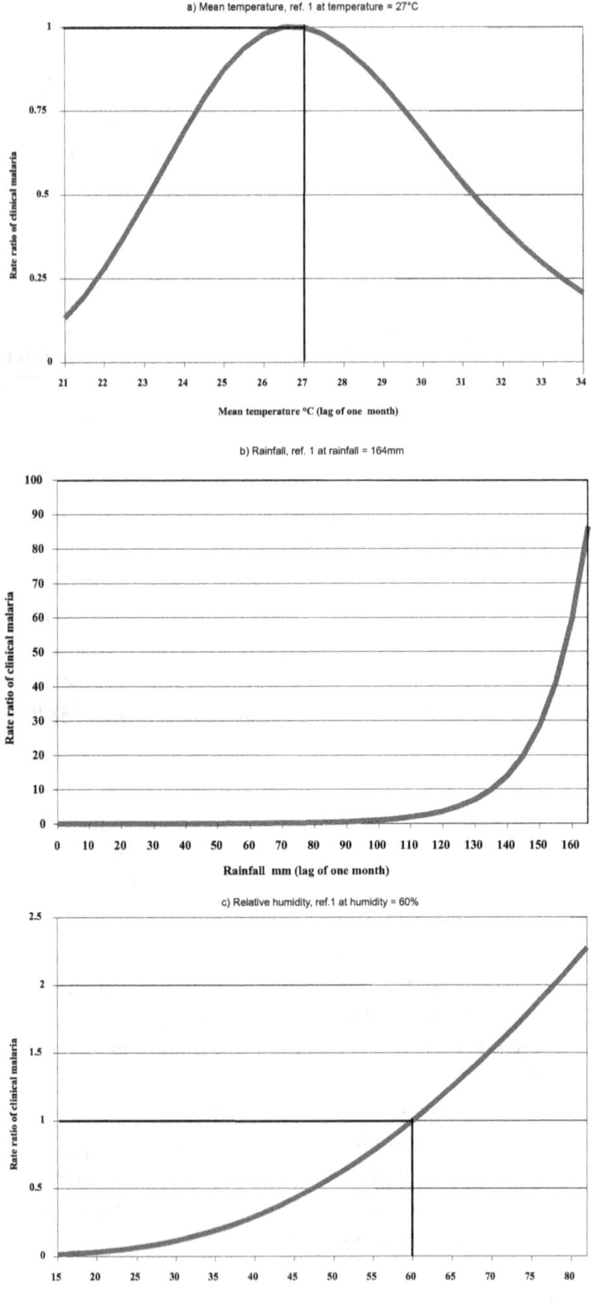

Figure 3.8 Impact of weather parameters on *P. falciparum* infection risk among study children, all sites combined

100 mm, the risk increased sharply and significantly for each increase of 10 mm of rain. For example the RR at 150 mm was 0.3 compared to 0.7 at 160 mm.

The RR for relative humidity was calculated using the 60% value as a reference point. This value corresponds to the minimum requirement for malaria vector development. Relative humidity observed in the field ranged from 15% to 80%. As the humidity increased, so did the risk of *P. falciparum* infection, but not in a linear form (Figure 3.8c). Below 60% of humidity there was a risk reduction. At 55% of relative humidity, the risk reduction was 25%. An exponential increase of *P. falciparum* infection risk was observed when the humidity was above 60%.

3.6 Mosquito population dynamics

3.6.1 Mosquito population abundance

3.6.1.1 Light Trap Capture A total of 96 LTC were performed in different houses in each site over 24 nights, giving an overall total of 384 LTCs. All species included, for all sites, 4,774 mosquitoes were caught. The largest proportion of captured mosquitoes was *Culex* (64.9%) followed by *An. Gambiae* (23.3%), *Mansonia* (7.6%), *An. Funestus* (4.0%), *An. nili* (0.23%) and *Aedes* (0.1%).

By site, the highest number of mosquitoes was caught in Nouna (47.5% of n=2,267), follow by Goni (27.3% of n=1,324), Cissé (14.1% of n=675) and Kodougou (10.6% of n=508). The distribution of mosquito species by site is shown in Figure 3.9. This figure has three dimensions. The mosquito species are shown on the X axis, the number of mosquitoes caught on the Y axis and the sites where mosquitoes were caught are shown on the Z axis. In all the sites, except Cissé, *Culex* mosquito was the most prominent species. However, in Nouna *Culex* represents a larger proportion of (88.0%) compared to Kodougou (52.2%) and Goni (44.3%). The number of *Culex* in Nouna was about two times more than the other three sites (1,997 vs. 1,003). The second most prominent specie was *An. Gambiae*. It represented 37.0% of the mosquitoes in Goni, 11.6% in Nouna: and 21.5% in Kodougou. In Cissé, *An. Gambiae* was more than the *Culex* (252 vs. 249). *Mansonia* and *An. funestus* were caught in Cissé, Goni and Kodougou. *An. nili* and *Aedes* were almost inexistent (Figure 3.9).

3.6.1.2 Human Land Capture 448 Human Land indoor and outdoor captures were performed over 14 nights in all the four sites. In each site, 112 captures were performed. 9,405 mosquitoes, all species included were caught. *Culex* mosquitoes, as in the LTC, were the dominant species (71.8%), followed by *An. gambiae* (13.5 %). In contrast to the LTC method, a significant number of *Aedes* mosquitoes were caught (9.3%). The largest proportion of mosquitoes was caught in Nouna (59.3%) where *Culex* is the most prominent species. The second largest proportion was caught in Goni (23.2%), followed by Cissé (12.1%) and Kodougou (5.4%). The

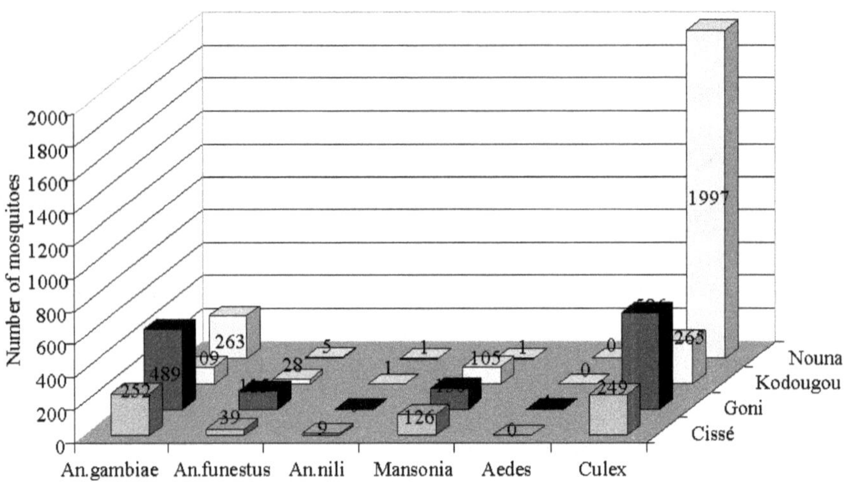

Figure 3.9 Distribution of mosquito species caught by LTC

distribution by species and sites (Figure 3.10) shows many *Culex* in Nouna and Goni. In all sites a significant number of *An. gambiae* were caught (Cissé: 346, Goni: 942, Kodougou: 174 and Nouna: 302). *Mansonia* and *Aedes* mosquitoes were caught in Cissé, Goni and Kodougou. In Cissé the *Aedes* represented 40.5% of the mosquitoes.

3.6.1.3 Pyrethrum Spray Capture 56 captures were performed over nine nights in each site. Overall, 2,923 mosquitoes were captured with a high proportion being caught in Nouna (35.9%) followed by Goni (26.7%), Cissé (20.7%) and Kodougou (26.0%). As in LTC and HLC, *Culex* mosquito (51.5%) was the most prominent species compared to *An. gambiae* (44.0%). While in Nouna and Cissé *Culex* mosquitoes were more than *An. gambiae*, in Goni and Kodougou it was the opposite. The highest number of *Mansonia* mosquitoes was caught in Cissé (67) (Figure 3.11).

In total, for all the three methods 20,593 mosquitoes were caught with the highest number being from HLC. The most prominent species was the *Culex* mosquito (68.0%) followed by *An. gambiae* (19.2%). The largest proportion of mosquitoes was caught in Nouna (11,083) compared to Goni (5,127) (Table 3.9).

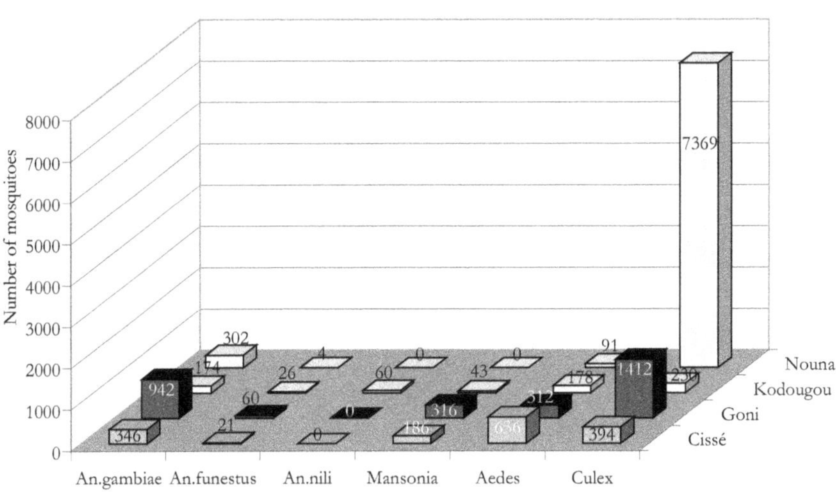

Figure 3.10 Distribution of mosquito species caught by HLC method

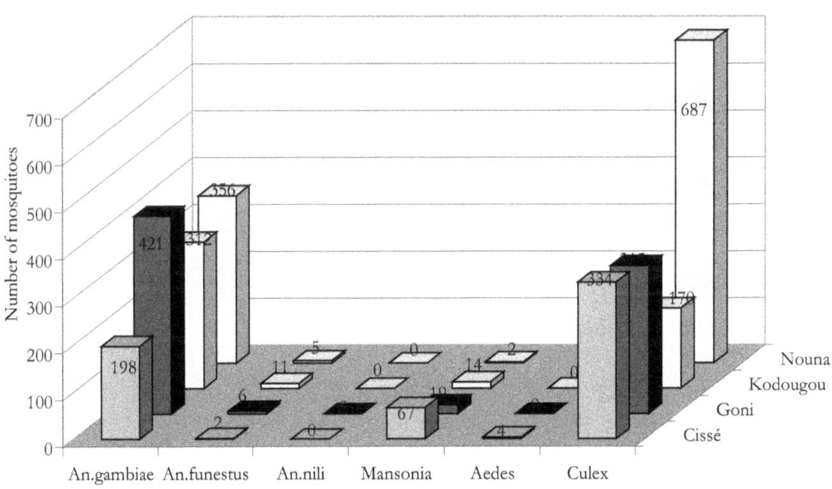

Figure 3.11 Distribution of mosquito species caught by PSC method

Table 3.9 Distribution of all mosquitoes caught by the three methods, site and species

		An.gambiae	*An.funestus*	*An.nili*	*Mansonia*	*Aedes*	*Culex*	*Total*
Cissé	N	796	62	9	379	640	977	2,863
	%	27.8	2.2	0.3	13.2	22.4	34.1	100
Goni	N	1,852	181	0	465	316	2,313	5,127
	%	36.1	3.5	0.0	9.1	6.2	45.1	100
Kodougou	N	400	65	61	162	178	665	1,531
	%	26.1	4.3	4.0	10.6	11.6	43.4	100
Nouna	N	921	14	1	3	91	10,053	11,083
	%	8.3	0.1	0.0	0.0	0.8	90.7	100
All	N	3,958	322	71	1,009	1,225	14,008	20,593
	%	19.2	1.6	0.3	4.9	6.0	68.0	100

In the following section we will look in more detail at the distribution of *An. gambiae* mosquitoes since it is the major malaria vector in this area.

3.6.2 An. gambiae abundance and distribution

Tables 3.10 and 3.11 give the monthly distribution of *An. gambiae* for each type of capture and by sites. In Table 3.10 the distribution is shown by place of capture (whether indoor or outdoor). The table shows the highest number of vectors was caught in August, September and October in all sites. The mean number of total vectors caught indoor (185.0) and outdoor (165.6) were not significantly different, (Student's paired t-test, two-tails distribution =0.12, p=0.09). There were no significant differences between mean numbers of mosquitoes caught indoor and outdoor in all the individual sites (t-test, Cissé: t=0.52, p=0.60, Goni: t=-0.18, p=0.85, Kodougou: t=0.66 p=0.51) despite the difference in values (Table 3.10). For indoor capture, the highest number of vectors was observed in Goni (438) and the lowest in Kodougou (110). A similar distribution was found in the outdoor capture (Table 3.10).

Table 3.10 HLC In and outdoor caught *An. gambiae* distribution, per site and month

	Indoor					Outdoor				
Month	Cissé	Goni	Kod*	Nouna	Total	Cissé	Goni	Kod*	Nouna	Total
Jan-04	0	2	0	0	2	1	0	0	2	3
Mar 04	0	0	4	0	4	0	0	2	0	2
May 04	0	0	3	0	3	0	0	1	1	2
Jul-04	0	15	0	1	16	3	1	0	0	4
Aug-04	178	155	51	16	400	83	252	17	17	369
Sep-04	22	211	44	118	395	14	168	38	118	338
Oct 04	23	55	8	15	101	22	83	6	14	125
Total	223	438	110	150	921	123	504	64	152	843
Mean	31.9	62.6	15.7	21.4	131.6	17.6	72.0	9.1	21.7	120.4
SD	65.3	86.0	22.0	43.2	185.0	30.1	101.9	14.1	43.0	165.6

* Kodougou

Table 3.11 shows the distribution of *An. gambiae* for LTC and PCS. The monthly trend is similar to the HLC. Consistently, in all sites vectors were more prominent in August, September and October. Few vectors were caught in December and November. In the other months there were practically no vectors; therefore, the monthly variation in vector number for all sites was very high, except Kodougou where it was relatively small (12.8). Goni remained the site with the highest number of vectors caught (LTC=489, PSC=421) (Table 3.11).

3.6.3 An. gambiae biting behaviour

An. gambiae biting activity is depicted in Figure 3.12. We observed that biting activity started slowly early in the evening (18:00 hours) and then increased progressively to reach a peak between 01:00 and 02:00 hours. From that time we observed a progressive drop until 0.5:00–06:00 hours. The biting activity was intense between 21:00 and 04:00 where more that 100 vectors were caught per hour. A drop was observed between 23:00 and 24:00.

3.6.4 An. gambiae population physiological age

An. gambiae caught were classified according to their physiological status (abdominal appearance). 52 mosquitoes were damaged during transportation and

Table 3.11 LTC and PSC *An. gambiae* caught distribution, per site and month

	LTC					PSC				
Month	Cissé	Goni	Kod*	Nouna	Total	Cissé	Goni	Kod*	Nouna	Total
Dec-03	9	21	24	5	59	–	–	–	–	–
Jan-04	4	1	2	0	7	–	–	–	–	–
Feb-04	4	0	7	0	11	–	–	–	–	–
Mar-04	0	0	0	0	0	–	–	–	–	–
Apr-04	0	0	1	2	3	–	–	–	–	–
May-04	0	0	0	0	0	–	–	–	–	–
Jun-04	0	2	3	0	5	–	–	–	–	–
Jul-04	1	12	0	2	15	–	–	–	–	–
Aug-04	190	142	15	53	400	93	0	10	68	171
Sep-04	21	231	41	188	481	80	248	45	196	569
Oct 04	18	77	16	12	123	25	173	62	92	352
Nov-04	5	3	0	1	9	–	–	–	–	–
Total	252	489	109	263	1113	198	421	117	356	1092
Mean	21.0	40.8	9.1	21.9	92.8	66.0	140.3	39.0	118.7	364.0
SD	53.7	73.9	12.8	54.4	167.1	–	–	–	–	–

*Kodougou

therefore could not be classified. The overall distribution is given in Figure 3.13. A large proportion (93.7%) of vectors caught by PSC method has completed their blood meal (fully fed, abdomen full of blood) and only 4.5% were gravid. Unfed vectors (had not taken a blood meal) were mainly caught by LTC (67.4%) and HLC (46.9%) methods. However, in both methods a significant proportion was fully fed. Semi-gravid and gravid vectors were mainly caught by HLC method where they represented respectively 13.8% and 19.6% of the vectors. Only a few vectors had not completed their blood meal.

3.6.4.1 An. gambiae gravid rate Monthly physiological status of the vector was assessed using the vectors caught by HLC method. In Table 3.12 the distribution of the vectors according to the physiological status is given by month and site. The proportion of gravid mosquitoes was also calculated. Semi-gravid and gravid vectors were pooled. Although the gravid rates were calculated for January and March, these results are not included in the description because the number of captured vectors was too small. Overall, the older vectors (semi-gravid and gravid) represented 33.4 % of the vectors caught. There were some differences between sites, with the

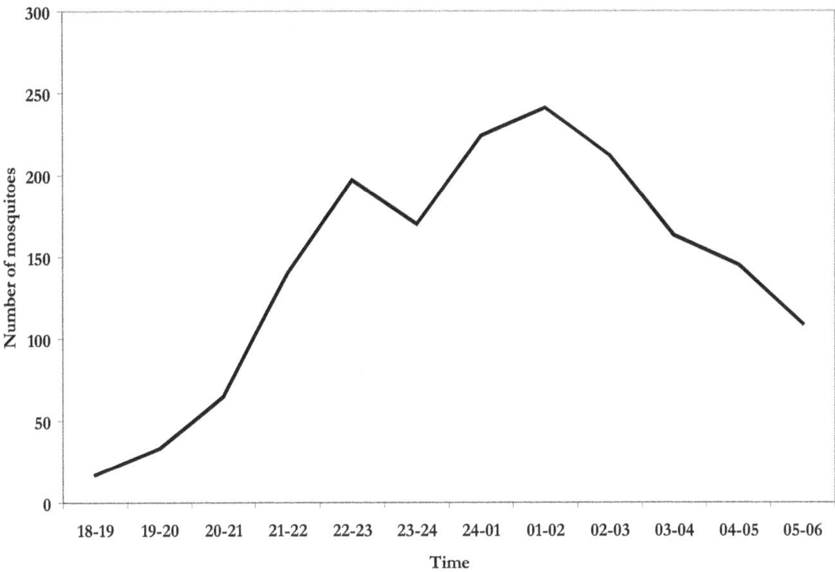

Figure 3.12 ***An. gambiae*** **human biting time (HLC)**

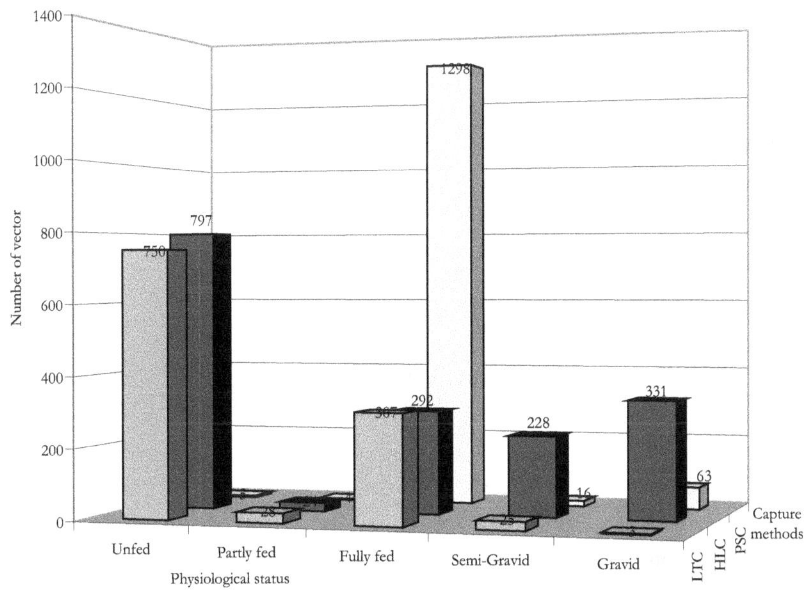

Figure 3.13 Overall distribution of *An. gambiae* according to their physiological status

Table 3.12 Distribution of *An. gambiae* vectors per site and by month according to their physiological age

Site	Month	Missing	Unfed	Partly fed	Fully fed	Semi gravid	Gravid	Total	Gravid %
All	Jan	2	1	1	0	0	1	5	33.3
	Mar	3	0	0	1	1	1	6	66.7
	Aug	46	308	15	79	124	188	760	43.7
	Sep	0	338	8	182	89	104	721	26.8
	Oct	1	150	0	30	14	37	232	22.1
	Total	52	797	24	292	228	331	1724	33.4
Cissé	Jan	1	0	0	0	0	0	1	0.0
	Mar	0	0	0	0	0	0	0	0.0
	Aug	0	92	7	43	62	57	261	45.6
	Sep	0	11	1	14	4	6	36	27.8
	Oct		23		7	3	12	45	33.3
	Total	1	126	8	64	69	75	343	42.1
Goni	Jan	0	1	0	0		1	2	50.0
	Mar	0	0	0	0	0	0	0	0.0
	Aug	41	157	8	30	52	113	401	45.8
	Sep	0	148	3	142	42	37	372	21.2
	Oct	0	95	0	18	7	18	138	18.1
	Total	41	401	11	190	101	169	913	31.0
Kodougou	Jan	0	0	0	0	0	0	0	0.0
	Mar	3	0	0	1	1	1	6	66.7
	Aug	4	42	0	6	7	6	65	21.3
	Sep	0	39	4	16	10	9	78	24.4
	Oct	1	17	0	1	0	2	21	10.0
	Total	8	98	4	24	18	18	170	22.2
Nouna	Jan	1	0	1	0	0	0	2	0.0
	Mar	0	0	0	0	0	0	0	0.0
	Aug	1	17	0	0	3	12	33	46.9
	Sep	0	140	0	10	33	52	235	36.2
	Oct	0	15	0	4	4	5	28	32.1
	Total	2	172	1	14	40	69	298	36.8

highest proportion in Cissé (42.1%), followed by Nouna (36.8%), Goni (31.0%) and Kodougou (22.2%). In all sites, August was consistently the month with the highest proportion of gravid vectors compared to September and October (Table 3.12).

3.6.4.2 An. gambiae parity rate The parity rate (proportion of vector which had oviposited at least once in their life) was assessed by dissection (see section 2.4.2.4). Only unfed *An. gambiae* mosquitoes caught by HLC method were considered. Table 20 gives the distribution by month and site of the proportion of parous vectors. Dissection was limited to the month with a significant number of mosquitoes. Overall, 33.9 % of the dissected *An. gambiae* were parous, with a significant difference across sites (Chi square test 13.9, p=0.0003). The largest proportion of parous vector was observed in Goni (38.5%) and Cissé (37.3%). In Kodougou (29.6%) and Nouna (23.3%) the rates were statistically similar to each other (Chi square test 1.3, p=0.25) and were below the overall rate. There were significant differences (Chi square 27.5, p=0.000) between months with a high rate observed in October consistently in all sites. Parous vectors were less common in August (Table 3.13).

Table 3.13 ***An. gambiae* caught by HLC method parity rate per month and sites**

Month	**Cissé**		**Goni**		**Kodougou**		**Nouna**		**All**	
	n	**Parous (%)**	**n**	**Parous (%)**	**n**	**Parous (%)**	**n**	**Parous (%)**	**n**	**Parous (%)**
Aug	92	27 (29.3)	157	45 (28.7)	42	8 (19.0)	17	7 (41.2)	308	87 (28.2)
Sept	11	6 (54.5)	148	62 (41.9)	39	13 (33.3)	140	24 (17.1)	338	105 (31.1)
Oct	23	14 (60.9)	95	47 (49.5)	17	8 (47.1)	15	9 (60.0)	150	78 (52.0)
Total	126	47 (37.3)	400	154 (38.5)	98	29 (29.6)	172	40 (23.3)	796	270 (33.9)

3.6.5 Comparing LTC and HLC indoor sampling of An. gambiae

The monthly total number for each site of *An. gambiae* mosquitoes caught by LTC method is compared to those caught indoor by HLC. HLC and LTC are correlated (Adjusted r^2=0.94). In Figure 3.14, a scatter plot with the fitted line, LTC (Y axis)

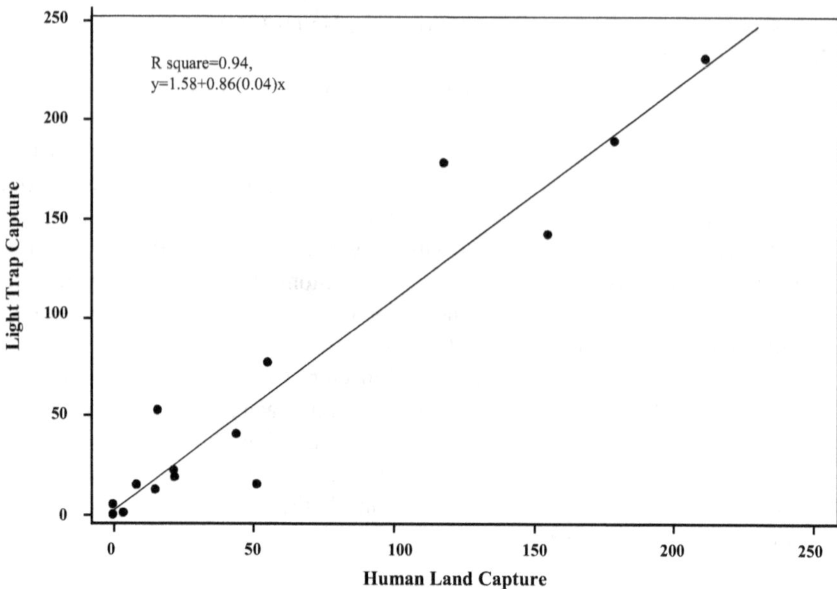

Figure 3.14 Scatter plot with regression line comparing number of vectors caught by LTC to those caught by HLC

is plotted against HLC (X axis). An increase in the number of vectors caught by HLC is highly associated with an increase of those caught by LTC.

3.6.6 An. gambiae mortality

An. gambiae generation mortality called *k-value* (expressed in log) was calculated monthly for each site. In Figure 3.15, the *k-value* is plotted per month. We observed very high and similar vector monthly mean mortality in all sites (Cissé: 2.0, Goni: 2.1, Kodougou: 2.1 and Nouna: 2.1). These *k-values* indicate a mortality of 99%. The figure shows a monthly fluctuation for all sites. The general pattern shows a significant decrease of the vector mortality from December to July where the mortality is lowest (Cissé: 0.83, Goni: 0.96, Kodougou: 0.80 and Nouna: 0.74) corresponding to mortality rates of 0.85, 0.89, 0.84 and 0.82 respectively. From July, the mortality rose and declined a bit earlier for Cissé (from August) and Nouna (from September), but later for Goni and Kodougou (from November).

When comparing the *k-value* with the expected vector abundance (estimated log of number of eggs) (Figure 3.16), we observed that in all sites, the mortality increased or decreased with the vector density. This relationship was better expressed from July onwards.

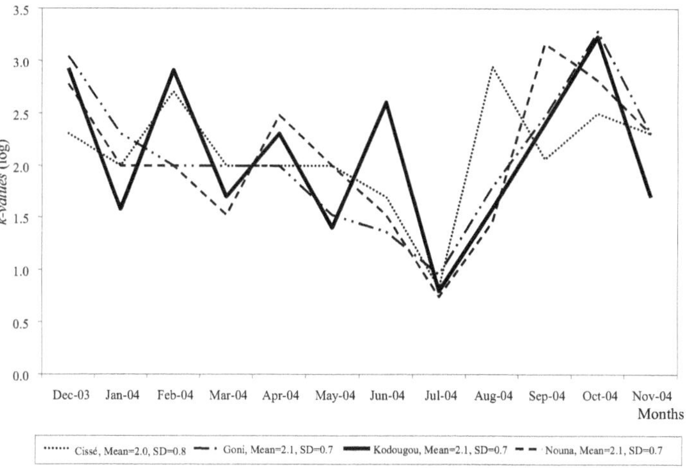

Figure 3.15 Monthly generation mortality (*k-value*) per site

The monthly average daily mortality rate of the vector was similar in all the sites with small variation over the year (Cissé: 0.15 SD: 0.04, Goni: 15 SD: 0.04; Kodougou: 0.15 SD: 0.05 and Nouna: 0.14 SD: 0.04). In all sites this rate was higher from May to June. In July, it decreased significantly and the lowest mortality rates were observed (Goni: 0.07, Cissé and Kodougou 0.06, Nouna: 0.05). From July to November the mortality rose again and remained above 0.10. Particularly high mortality rates (above 0.20) were observed in the September, October and February (Figure 3.17).

3.6.7 An. gambiae sporogonic cycle

The sporogonic cycle duration express the time in days needed for the parasite to complete its development in the vector host. This duration is temperature-dependent and is calculated using Detinova 1962 formula (c=111/T°C-18) described in detail in the methods section. The sporogonic cycle duration influences the vectorial capacity. It was calculated by site and by month given the average temperature. On average, the cycle takes about the same time in all the sites (Cissé: 10.6 days SD: 2.7; Goni: 13.3 SD: 6.8, Kodougou: 11.7 SD: 3.4 and Nouna: 9.9 SD: 1.9). However, it was slightly longer in Goni. We observed the duration varied over the year, with the shortest period observed in April and May (7 days). These months correspond to the hottest period in the year. From March to November there were no significant differences across sites, whereas in December and February the differences were pronounced. The cycle was particularly long in Goni in December, ten days longer than the other sites (Figure 3.18).

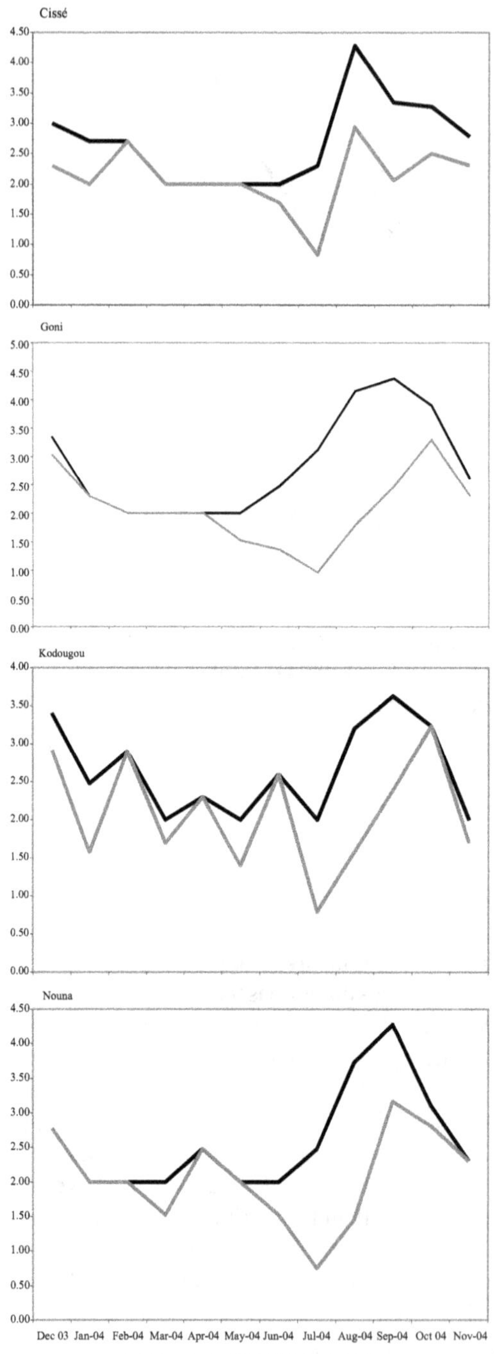

Figure 3.16
***An. gambiae* density-dependent generation mortality (*k-value*)**

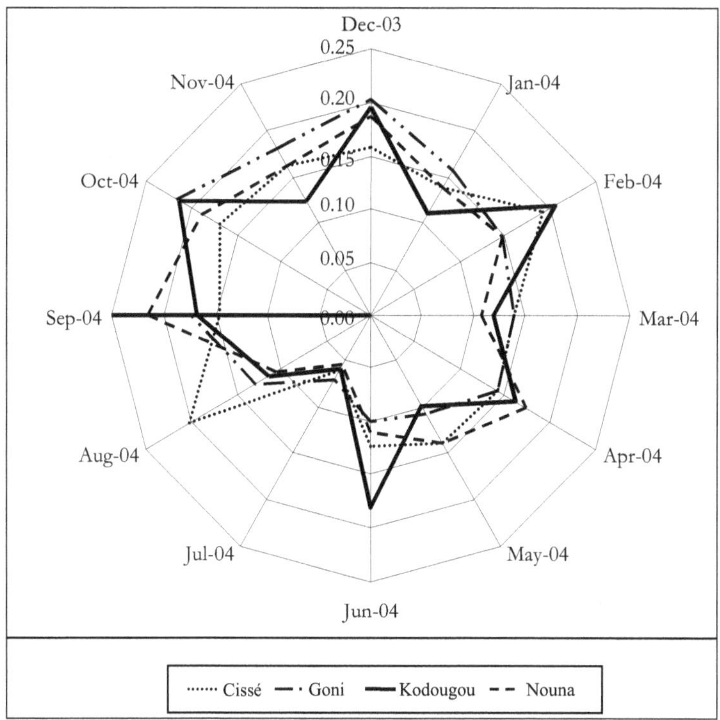

Figure 3.17 Spider diagram of *An. gambiae* daily mortality rate

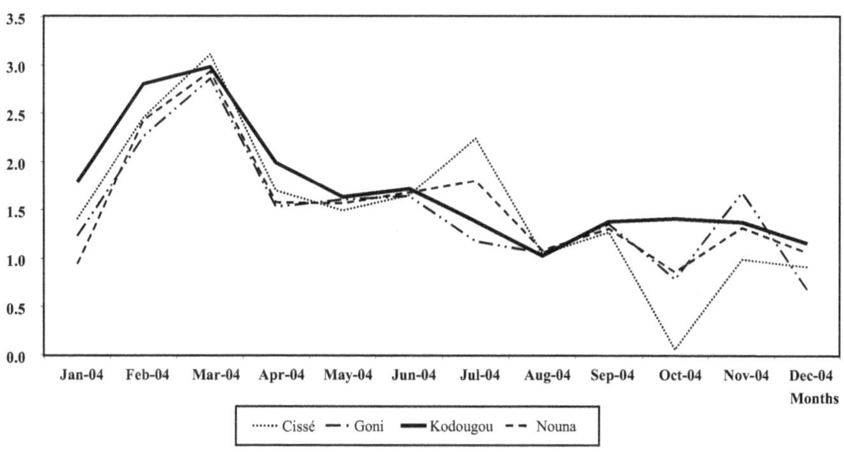

Figure 3.18 Monthly variation of the sporogonic cycle duration in days

3.6.8 An. gambiae vectorial capacity

The daily Vectorial Capacity (VC) which is defined as the expected inoculations of human per infective case per time unit was calculated for each individual site. Figure 3.19 shows a monthly plot of the VC in each site on a logarithmic scale. In Goni, we observed the highest average VC with the highest variation over the year (43.8, SD: 74.0), followed by Nouna (23.9, SD: 43.4), Cissé (14.5, SD: 22.2) and Kodougou (9.4, SD: 11.1) where the lowest VC was observed. There was a significantly high variation for all sites over the year, which was particularly high in Goni. Figure 3.19 shows a progressive increase of the VC from December to August where the peak values were observed in all the sites. From August there was rapid decrease for all sites except Kodougou where it remained similar in September. In October and November the VC dropped consistently. From May to October the highest VC was observed in Goni and the lowest in Kodougou. The VC was particularly low in Goni in December, January and February.

3.6.9 An. gambiae human biting rate and EIR

An. gambiae daily human biting rate, expressing the number of bites a person received per night was calculated using mosquitoes captured by HLC. The monthly specific daily rates were obtained by dividing the number of vectors caught by eight (number of persons involved in the capture) and by two (number of nights of capture). The annual rates were obtained by multiplying the total daily rates by 365.25. The total daily rates were calculated by dividing the total number of

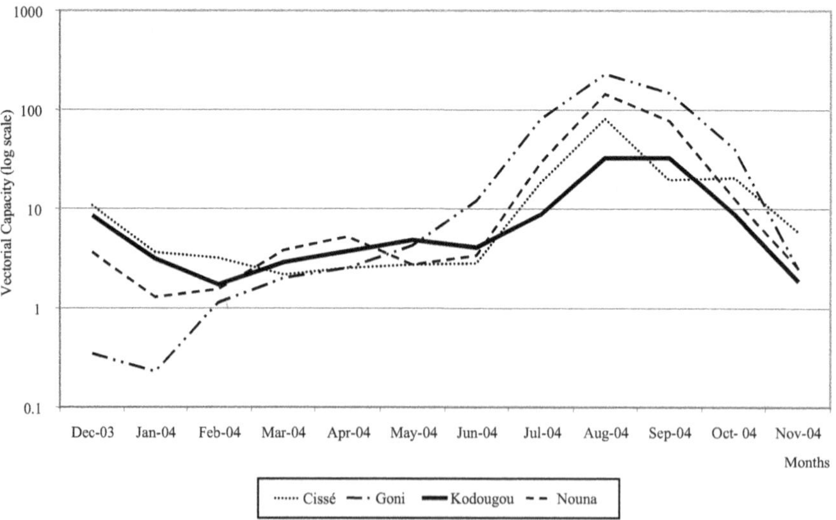

Figure 3.19 Estimation of *An. gambiae* daily vectorial capacity

vectors (caught over the seven months) by 56 (total number of persons involved in the capture) and by 14 (total number of nights). The month and site specific biting rates are presented in Table 3.14.

In all sites from January to July people got less than one bite per night. In August the number of bites increased substantially in Goni (25.4 bites) and Cissé (16.3 bites), while in Kodougou and Nouna it remained relatively low. In September a significant decrease was observed in Cissé (2.3), but an increase was observed in Nouna (14.8). In Goni and Kodougou the number of bites remained about the same as in September. For all sites a significant decrease was observed in October. The people in Goni altogether got 438.3 nightly bites in a year, five times more than those living in Kodougou (80.4 bites), three times more than those in Nouna (142.5 bites) and 2.7 times more those in Cissé (160.7 bites) (Table 3.14).

Table 3.14 Monthly *An. gambiae* human biting rates per site, based on human land capture

Months	Cissé	Goni	Kodougou	Nouna	All
Jan	0.1	0.1	0	0.13	0.1
Mar	0.0	0.0	0.4	0.0	0.1
May	0.0	0.0	0.3	0.1	0.1
Jul	0.2	1.0	0.0	0.1	0.3
Aug	16.3	25.4	4.3	2.1	12.0
Sep	2.3	23.7	5.1	14.8	11.5
Oct	2.8	8.6	0.9	1.8	3.5
Total	0.4	1.2	0.2	0.4	0.6
Annual bite/person/night	160.7	438.3	80.4	142.5	204.5

Compared to the biting rate the entomological inoculation rate (EIR) was low. It expresses the number of infective bites a person gets per night over a defined period of time, usually one year. In Table 3.15, for each individual month and site the daily infective bites rates and the annual rates are given based on the daily total rate. For all the three months, people in Goni received the highest infective bites per night compared to the other sites. The numbers were above two bites per night. The annual rates for Goni were significantly higher compared to Kodougou where the lowest rate was observed (58.3). In Cissé, the highest daily rate was observed in August (1.7), while in Nouna it was in September (1.6). The overall monthly rates are about the same and annual rate was 333.8 bites per night, three times higher than the individual site rates of Cissé (119.2) and Nouna (104.0) (Table 3.15).

Table 3.15 Number of infected bites per person per night

Month	Cissé	Goni	Kodougou	Nouna	All
Aug	1.7	2.8	0.5	0.4	1.3
Sep	0.4	3.9	0.6	1.6	1.6
Oct	0.9	2.9	0.3	0.6	1.2
Total	0.3	1.1	0.2	0.3	0.5
Annual EIR	119.2	388.1	58.3	104.0	167.4

3.7 Weather-based dynamic model of malaria transmission

3.7.1 Prediction of An. gambiae population

The effect of temperature and rainfall on *An. gambiae* population density was assessed by a dynamic model (described in detail in section 2.7.4). The model, driven by rainfall and temperature was simulated independently for each site except Kodougou where rainfall data was missing. The model parameter values are described in table (Table 3.16) while the parameters descriptions are given in the methods section (Table 2.7).

Table 3.16 Model parameter values and bounds

Parameters	Cissé[bounds]	Gon[bounds]	Nouna[bounds]
α	0.000126	0.000126	0.000126
β_1	0.000096	0.000096	0.000096
β_2	0.000041	0.000041	0.000041
q	0.12 [0.10–0.17]	0.12 [0.10–0.17]	0.12 [0.10–0.17]
v	10 days [9–15]	10 days [9–15]	10 days [9–15]
r	2	2	2
m	0.15 [0.06–0.20]	0.15 [0.07–0.22]	0.14[0.05–0.22]
b	0.56 [0.5–0.6]	0.56 [0.5–0.6]	0.56 [0.5–0.6]
γ	0.79	0.79	0.79
c	10.6 days [9–14]	13.3 days [9–14]	9.9 days [9–14]

The model simulation outputs are depicted for each site in Figure 3.20. The simulated *An. gambiae* population is plotted with the daily temperature and previous two week cumulative rainfall. The left Y axis (on logarithmic scale) represents the number of predicted vector numbers; the right one represents the temperature (in °C) and the rainfall (in mm). The X axis represents the time in days. The simulation was done daily for two years (2004 and 2005). The year 2004 was considered as a training (warm-up) period of the model. As temperature and rainfall data for the year 2005 were not yet available, the conditions were assumed to be similar to 2004; therefore, temperature and rainfall were replicated. In all the three sites, rainfall was followed by an increase in the mosquito population two weeks later. The impact of mean temperature was small.

In Cissé, we observed that mosquitoes were few (less that ten a day) in the first 120 days of the year, corresponding to the months from January to May. In this period there was no rainfall observed. The first peak of mosquito numbers was observed in the 122nd day of the year, followed by a second one a month later. These peaks were all observed after a peak of rainfall. Two other peaks of mosquito's abundance were observed one month after the second peak. This increase corresponded to July and August, months with high rainfall. From August, the vector population decreased significantly toward the end of year, after the offset of the rainfall.

In Goni, the simulation showed several peaks of vector population following by each peak of rainfall. Like in Cissé, these peaks were clustered within a period from the 121st to 301st days of the year. This period corresponds to that between May and October. In contrast to Cissé, although we saw some daily fluctuation, the vector population remained relatively high over this period, probably because of the relative high rainfall. After the offset of the rainfall, we observed a drop of the mosquito population.

Nouna site has about the same pattern of mosquito's abundance and distribution as in Goni, although, the rainfall was more abundant. The mosquito population increased shortly after the onset of the rainfall. It remained high (about 100 a day), with some fluctuation, until the stop of the rainfall where there was a decrease up to less than ten mosquitoes a day. As in the two other sites the highest peak of the mosquito's population was observed about two weeks after the highest peak of rainfall in August.

In Figure 3.21, the monthly prediction (broken line) of *An. gambiae* is compared to those caught in the field (full line). The Y axis represents the number of vectors and the X axis the months.

The model prediction showed a peak of vector numbers for all sites in September, matching with the observation for Goni and Nouna. In Cissé the peak of caught mosquito numbers was observed one month earlier in August and therefore, did not match with the prediction. Consistently in all sites the model prediction matched with the observed from January to April (few numbers). In June, in Cissé and Goni, the prediction showed an increase in mosquito population which was not observed in the field. In all three sites there was a significant decline

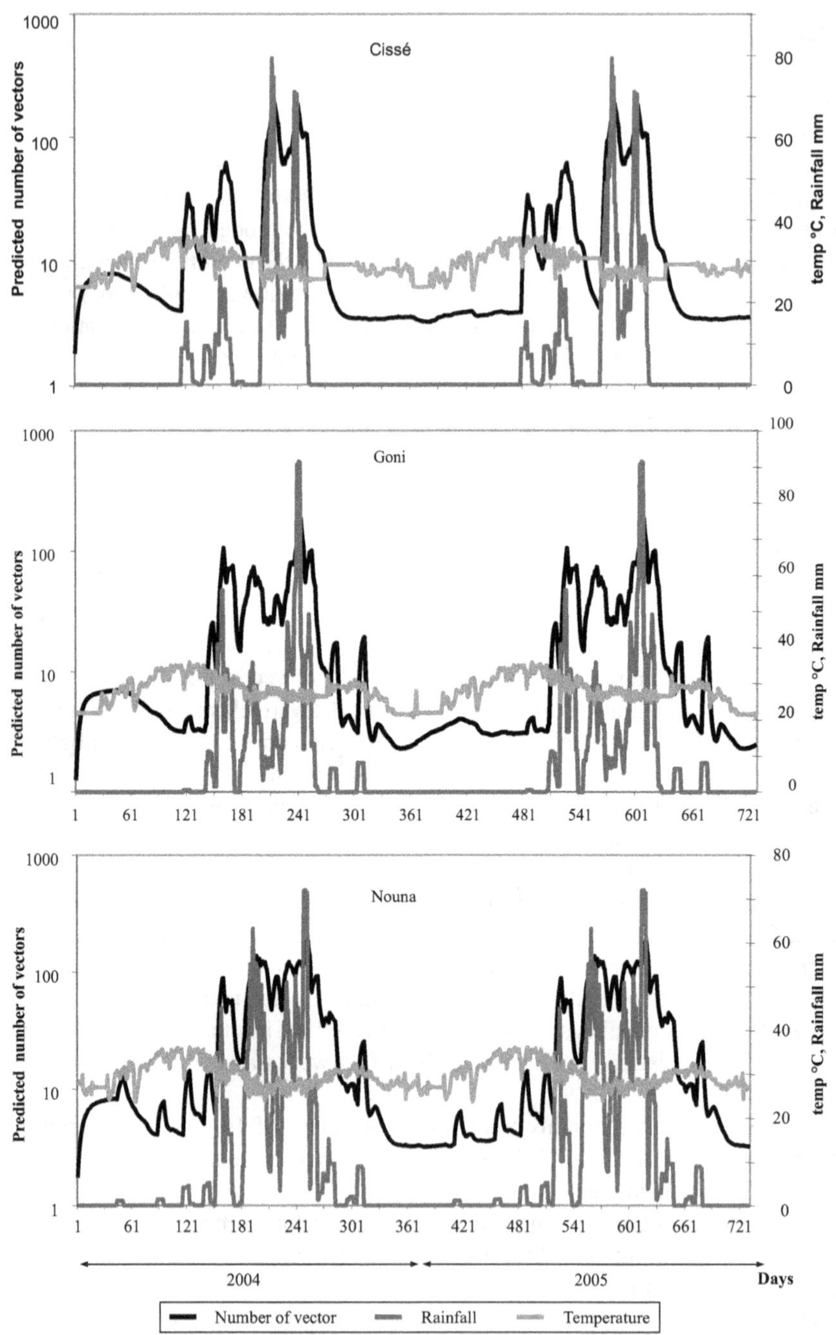

Figure 3.20 Mean temperature and rainfall based prediction of *An. gambiae* population abundance

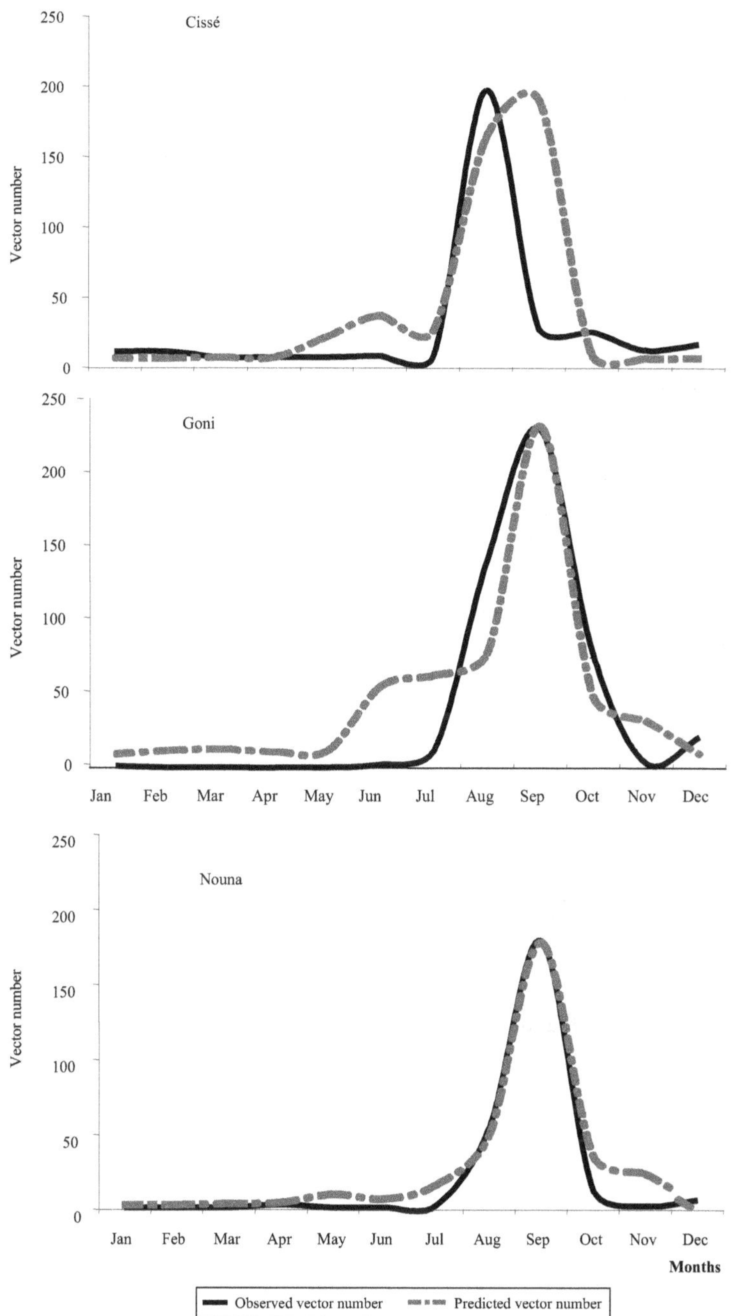

Figure 3.21 Predicted monthly *An. gambiae*, compared to observed for each site

(prediction and observed) of the vector population in October and both remained low in November and December.

Overall, the model predictions followed a similar pattern as the observed. The fit was better in Nouna where we observed the least variance ($\Delta = \sum (O_i - P_i)^2 =$ 1696.5, SD=8.8), Where O_i is the observed number of the vector population in the month and P_i the predicted number from the model. The variances for Goni and Cissé were 11630.4 and 35292.2 respectively.

3.7.2 Prediction of human infection

P. falciparum infection incidence cases among children were also simulated by the model per site and per month. The model values remained the same as preliminary calculated and fitted (See section 3.7.1). The predicted cases (normalised) were compared to the observed ones and variances ($\Delta = \sum (O_i - P_i)^2$) were estimated. Figure 3.22 shows the plot of the predicted cases (broken line) and the observed (full line) plus the 95% confidence limits, CI (vertical lines) for each monthly predicted value. They define the prediction range of the model given an error (α) of 5%. CI was calculated with the following formula, $95\%CI = P_i \pm 1.96 * SE$ where P_i is the predicted value of a particular month and SE the standard error of the predicted value for each observed.

For all sites, there was a seasonal pattern of the *P. falciparum* infection incidence. This was shown by the prediction and the observed cases. From December to June the incidences decreased progressively then increased from July to September. At this point in time another decrease was observed. Although the general patterns of the prediction and observed were similar (the 95% CI of the prediction included in most cases the observed value), there were some specific variations expressed by the variance Δ. The model prediction match better with the observed for Goni where the least variance was observed (Δ=626.8 SE=6.6), compared to Nouna (Δ=733.7, SE=4.8) and Cissé (Δ=882.8, SD=6.7).

For all sites the model could not capture the increase of cases observed in March, probably due to that fact this corresponds to the dry period, and the model was driven by rainfall and temperature.

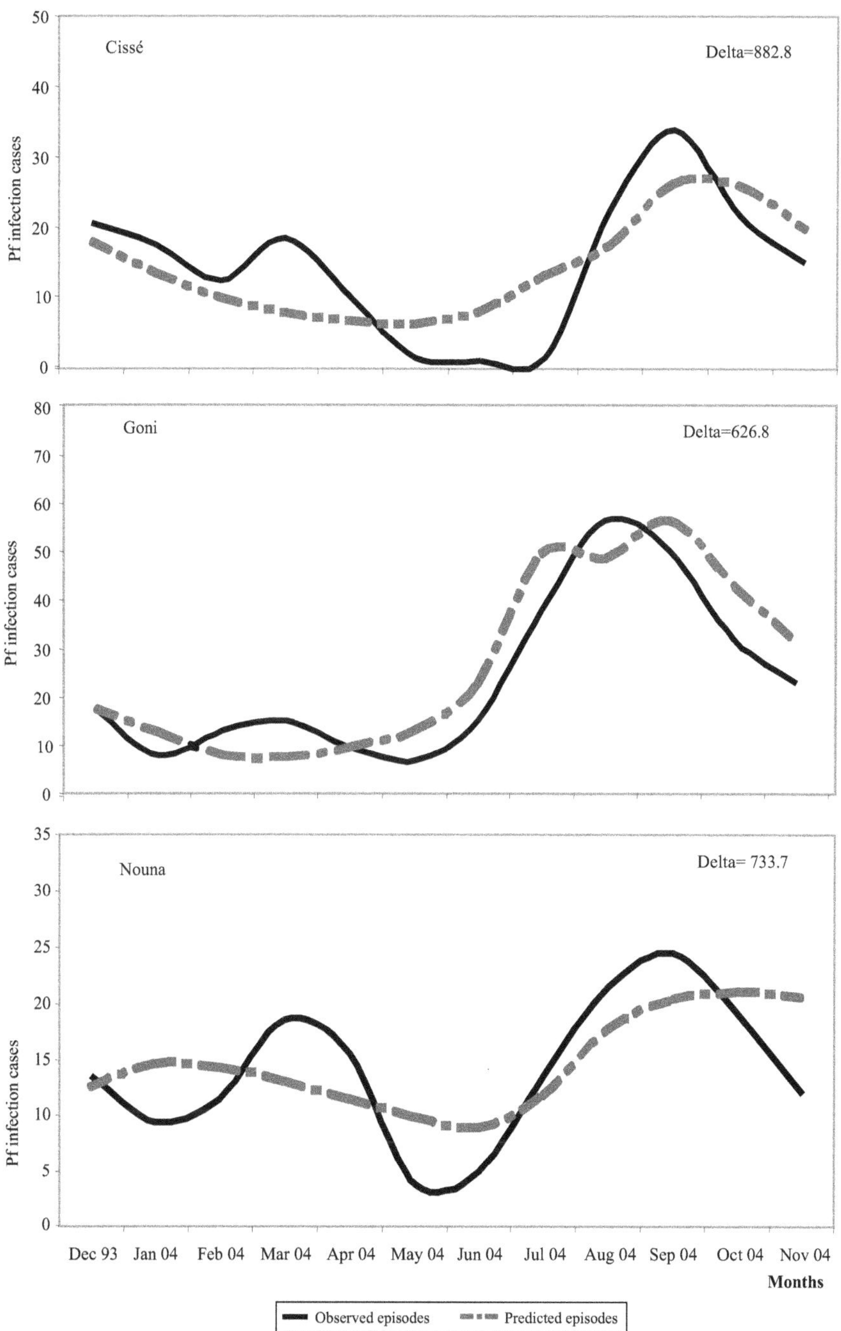

Figure 3.22 Predicted monthly *P. falciparum* infection cases compared to observed ones for each site

Chapter 4
Discussion and Conclusions

This chapter will be divided into two major subchapters: the discussion and conclusions. In this first section, we will discuss the findings according to the study questions and objectives, and also the response rate. Then, each individual objective will be discussed. The first subchapter will end by discussing the limitations observed at each level: design, data collection and analysis, how they were mitigated and how they may affect the findings. The second subchapter will be dedicated to the possible public health impact of the findings and some recommendations. These recommendations will be made for both malaria scientists and decision makers.

4.1 Discussion

4.1.1 P. falciparum infection survey

4.1.1.1 Study population characteristics The study population characteristics were identical in all the sites. Indeed, the sex and age distribution were not statistically different across sites. This suggests a good sampling procedure. The study was limited to 6 to 59 months, because of their particular susceptibility to *P. falciparum* malaria infection (Lusingu et al. 2004, Reyburn et al. 2005, Shanks et al. 2005). Children below 6 months are less susceptible due to maternal protection. This immunity is progressively lost with age, and a child, by being exposed to mosquito bites develops his own immunity, which is relatively stronger after his fifth year. However, this acquired immunity will not protect him from *P. falciparum* infection, but from developing clinical symptom of malaria. This scenario is typical in areas where malaria is endemic.

Ethnic group distribution was different between sites. This was expected as people settle according to their social belonging; therefore, in the rural settings, villages are mainly inhabited by one ethnic group. This is the case in Cissé where most children are Fulani, Goni (Marka) and Kodougou (Mossi). Because Nouna is a semi-urban settlement, all the ethnic groups in the district were represented. Ethnicity was considered as a proxy for genetic susceptibility. Some studies have reported the Fulani ethnic group to been less susceptible to malaria compared to the others (Modiano et al. 1996, 1998).

Starting with 867 children, the follow up attained an excellent retention rate (96.8%), which was achieved because of the clear identification of the children provided by the DSS in place and less mobility of the study population. As expected at the end of the follow up, the age structure was significantly different across sites. Sex and ethnic distribution remained the same as the children lost to follow up were almost equally distributed across sites by these covariates.

4.1.1.2 Response rate Although this was an intensive survey, the overall weekly response rate was good 87.7%. We have made a distinction between loss to follow up and non-response. While the first one is defined as children who have left the observation by out migration or death, the second one is described as the absence during a particular visit. This can be because of travel, referral to hospital or temporary out migration. The high response rate could be explained by the close contact of the interviewers with the family, but mainly by treatment provided for sick children. This aspect was well appreciated by the community.

A low response rate was observed during the rainy season (Figure 3.2) due to farming activities. In this period mothers have to go farming for the whole day. Some even stay in the fields during the whole farming season, which lasts from June to October. The relatively low response rate of Nouna is attributed to its semi-urban status. Mothers are involved in small trading activities, and therefore, are not always available. The response rate was particularly high in Goni, probably because of the predominance of the ethnic group Marka. The Marka are culturally known to be more receptive than Fulani and Mossi, maybe because of this social organisation. Marka, are part of the so-called unorganised community, without any strong hierarchical structure. Households are therefore free to make their own decisions. In contrast, Mossi and Fulani have high hierarchical social structures where decisions are made by a chief. In case of no involvement of the chief's family in a study, the community is always sceptical. Another possible explanation for high response rate in Goni could be fact that the interviewer was from this village. These differences in response rate between sites did not affect the results of the study.

4.1.2 Weather changes and P falciparum infection among U5 at small-scale level (Study question 1)

4.1.2.1 P. falciparum infection risk according to ecological settings (Objective 1) A high incidence of fever was observed in all the four sites with no significant difference. Overall, an average of two episodes per child per year was reported. This high incidence corroborates with findings by Müller et al. (2001). The origin of these fevers is not totally attributable to malaria infection. Only half of them tested *P. falciparum* positive. This pattern was consistent in all sites. This suggests that fever alone is not sensitive enough for malaria detection as shown also by Dicko et al. (2005).

Overall in the individual sites, the *P. falciparum* infection incidence was high. We observed at least one episode per child per year in the rural sites. In Nouna it was relatively low at 0.5 episodes per child per year. The high number of episodes observed in Goni and Kodougou could be because of their ecological settings.

Goni is located in a plain where there is seasonal practice of rice farming which creates mosquito habitats. Kodougou is a village near (200 meters) a perennial river, by which traditional irrigated farming takes place. Proximity to irrigated and flooded agriculture practices have been reported to be highly associated with malaria infection (Baldet et al. 2003, Sissoko et al. 2004, Koudou et al. 2005). The particular low incidence of *P. falciparum* infection (two times less than in the other sites) reported in Nouna is probably attributable to the semi-urban setting. Urban settings are reported to be less malaria prone compared to rural settings (Omumbo et al. 2005) because of the pollution of water bodies which are then unsuitable for the malaria vector.

Clinical malaria episodes defined as fever plus *P. falciparum* density of>=5000/μ/l, in line with Müller et al. (2001), were also very high in all sites; about one episode per child per year. This was a surprising result, as we were expecting fewer episodes because of the treatment provided. There are two possible explanations. First the non-response of children to the Chloroquine treatment because of resistance of the parasite, already reported to be high in this area. Indeed, Müller et al. (2004) reported a community based Chloroquine treatment failure of 33%. The second explanation may be the difference in case definitions. We did not include a window period from one episode to another. Müller et al. (2001) had a window period of 20 days, whereby a new episode was considered only 20 days after the previous one. In our case every positive test was considered to be a new episode; therefore, the same episode may have persisted the following week and been counted as a new episode.

Severe malaria episodes, defined as *P. falciparum* density of =>100, 000/μ/l (Mueller et al. 2001), were few probably due to treatment provided, which was able to reduce the parasite load.

P. falciparum infection and clinical malaria were highly seasonal in all sites. The highest number of cases was observed in August, September and October (Figure 3.4). These months correspond to the rainy season. Rainfall creates breeding sites for the vector, thereby increasing their population, and hence the number of human-vector contacts. The high number of cases in December is driven by residual mosquitoes from the rainy season or new incoming mosquitoes from the remaining breeding sites. The sudden drop of cases in January consistently in all sites is probably the result of the drop in temperature resulting in a slow development process of the vector. The increase of temperature in February and March resulted in an increase of the number of cases, although there was no rainfall. This is what we called ‘dry season malaria’, suggesting there are still some breeding sites available. These could be human-made, like the surroundings of wells or irrigated vegetable gardens common in this area. In this period because of the high temperature the development process of the vector is short; therefore, even short lasting water bodies could be enough for the vector to complete its development cycle. From April, the high temperature could have resulted in very high evaporation and an increase of the vector mortality leading to dramatic decrease of the *P. falciparum* infection cases.

Two modelling approaches have been used to assess the risk of *P. falciparum* infection among children given their site of residence, taken as an ecological setting. The first model (called model A) is a conventional binary response logistic regression model, and the second one (Model B) is also a logistic model, which however integrates three levels random effects (Mauny et al. 2004).

- **Model A**

  According to Model A, children living in Kodougou and Goni are more likely to be *P. falciparum* infection positive compared to those living in Nouna (Urban setting). This could be explained by reasons already discussed above. These two sites are located respectively in a plain and near a perennial river. Farming practices next to the river creates a conducive environment for malaria vectors. Other covariates included in the model showed different effects on the odds for *P. falciparum* infection.

  Older children were better protected compared to the young ones. The odds are much higher in the age group below 12 months. This can be explained by the loss of partial immunity gained from the mother, which lasts for about six months after birth. Reyburn et al. (2005) reported high odds of severe malaria in the age group below 12 months. With the increase of age, children develop their partial immunity and become less susceptible, although below five years this immunity remains weak.

  Ethnicity has been suggested to play a role in genetic susceptibility where the Fulani are less susceptible compared to others (Modiano et al. 1996, 1999). However, our findings did not confirm this. We found the odds of *P. falciparum* infection of Mossi, Samo, Marka and Bwaba to be statistically similar to those of the Fulani (Peuhl). Studies specifically designed to explore this association in this region maybe of interest, as understanding genetic susceptibility to *P. falciparum* infection could be useful for vaccine development.

  Self-reported mosquito net use was surprisingly not associated with a decrease in *P. falciparum* infection risk among children as has been extensively reported in other studies (Hawley et al. 2003, Lengeler 2004). The question was precise enough to get the real information as described in the methods section. Mothers were asked at each visit whether the child had been sleeping under a mosquito net since the preceding visit. Though, distinction was made between normal mosquito nets and insecticide-treated nets (ITN) for the data collection, this was not considered in the analysis. This was because of the very small number of non-impregnated mosquito nets, as ITN were given free in the framework of an ongoing trial project. This result could be explained by our case definition (Fever + presence of any number of parasites). Even children using mosquito nets are exposed to vector bites, which start at 19.00 hours (Figure 3.13), when children are not yet under the mosquito net.

Children who had received treatment during the previous visit were less likely to be tested positive. This result suggested some protection of the Chloroquine treatment, despite the high resistance reported in some studies (Müller et al. 2003).

Among the housing condition factors, only the presence of farming activities within 30 metres radius from the household was associated with increased odds of *P. falciparum* infection. This could be explained by the presence of small pools of water created within the crop by digging. The agriculture practice in this region is to make small furrows between the crops to retain rainfall water for better ground infiltration. Such water bodies combined with the shadow provided by the crops create a suitable environment for vector breeding; therefore, increasing the risk of *P. falciparum* infection. The observed reduction in odds for children living in brick houses is similar to what has been observed in other studies (Gamage-Mendis et al. 1991, Lindsay et al. 2003, Palsson et al. 2004), though the OR were not statistically significant. This could be explained by the homogenous situation of houses in this area. Indeed, 95% of the houses are traditionally made of mud blocks assumed to be less well-constructed compared to the brick ones. We therefore had too few children living in brick houses to yield statistical significance, although we observed a reduction of 0.6 in the odds of *P. falciparum* infection for children living in brick houses.

The rainy season, as expected is highly associated with an increase of *P. falciparum* infection cases. In this region of dry climate, breeding sites (open water bodies) for malaria vector are mainly provided by rainfall, occurring mainly during a specific period of the year. In contrast, during the dry season, the hot and dry weather is less suitable for vectors, therefore leading to high vector mortality and reduction in infection. This finding is consistent with other studies (Dicko et al. 2005, Shililu et al. 2004).

- **Model B**

  After controlling for individual and household level variation, the effect of site of residence on *P. falciparum* infection odds was cancelled. This suggests that, Model A was not able to assess the influence of the individual child and household factors on the odds of *P. falciparum* infection given the available covariates. Individual biological factors (except age) or genetic susceptibility were not measured in the field; therefore, not included in the model. It is known that children have different genetic susceptibilities (Ruwende et al. 1995, May and Horstmann 2004). Similarly, it was not feasible to collect data on all possible household factors that could influence the malaria transmission among children. For example, household economic status data were not collected, yet is known to contribute to malaria prevention and treatment seeking behaviour, and vary from one household to another (Biritwum et al. 2000, Uzochukwu and Onwujekwe 2004).

As shown by the variance estimate, there is heterogeneity in the probability of being *P. falciparum* positive between individual children and within households. This variability is because of but by unknown or unmeasured variables (Mauny et al. 2004). The random effects can therefore be considered as a composite of unknown or unmeasured individual and household factors influencing the probability of *P. falciparum* infection (Goldstein and Rasbash 1996).

In conclusion, the four sites considered as different ecological settings have the same odds of *P. falciparum* infection, when considering, all the individual and household factors which vary across sites.

4.1.2.2 Effect of weather of P. falciparum infection risk (Objective 2) Weather parameters are known to be important predictors for *P. falciparum* infection as already discussed in the previous sections. However, the individual effect of each parameter varies. We explored individual effects with interaction terms between mean temperature, rainfall and relative humidity of the previous month on *P. falciparum* infection risk among children in the three sites where rainfall data were available. In addition, we also assessed the combined effect of "temperature-rainfall", "temperature-relative humidity" and "rainfall-relative humidity".

Mean temperature alone was a strong predictor for *P. falciparum* infection among children. Its relationship with *P. falciparum* infection is "bell-shaped" (Figure 3.9). Low and high temperatures reduce *P. falciparum* infection risk. The infection risk is optimal at medium temperature, around 27°C. At mean temperatures of 23°C and 31°C the risk reduction compared to 27°C is about 50%. There is no direct biological link between human infection and ambient temperature. However, these results can be explained by the temperature-dependence of the vector life cycle. Indeed, it has been demonstrated that the sporogonic cycle (the development of the parasite) is shorter (9–10 days) at temperature of 28°C and longer (about 100 days) at temperature below 20°C (Macdonald 1957, Bradley et al. 1987). Therefore, a short incubation period allows the vector to live long enough to become infectious and transmit the infection. The lifespan of the vector is about 21 days. At high temperatures the vector survival decreases. A temperature of 40°C will result in 0% of survival. The combination of the sporogonic cycle and the vector survival gives the vector surviving sporogeny expressing the proportion of vectors surviving the incubation period. Craig et al. (1999) reported it to be high at temperatures between 28°C and 32°C. This supports our results since at this temperature one would expect many infectious vectors to cause an increase of *P. falciparum* infection incidence. In all the sites we found the mean annual temperature to be 28°C, justifying the high incidence in *P. falciparum* infection. In addition, a temperature above 27°C increases the feeding frequency (etwo days) of the vector as the blood digestion rate increases. This results in more frequent vector-human contact. Our findings are in line with several other studies (Kleinschmidt et al. 2001a, Shanks et al. 2002, Teklehaimanot et al. 2004).

The cumulative rainfall of the preceding month had a positive effect on *P. falciparum* infection. Similar results of positive effect of rainfall on malaria have been consistently reported by several studies (Lindsay and Martens 1998, Lindblade et al. 1999, Githeko abd Ndegwa 2001, Teklehaimanot et al. 2004, Zhou et al. 2005). The relationship is "J" shape, suggesting a non-linear relationship contrary to Teklehaimanot et al. (2004) and suggesting that a minimum threshold quantity of rainfall is necessary for transmission to take place. A minimum of 100 mm was necessary to observe an increase of *P. falciparum* infection rate. This threshold could be explained by the hot and dry climate leading to very high evaporation and infiltration, resulting in non availability of surface water for vector breeding. Small amounts of rainfall will evaporate or infiltrate in a shorter time, while with high levels of rainfall, some water remains long enough for the vector to complete the development cycle. At a higher level (160mm), an increase of rainfall has very little effect on the *P. falciparum* infection, suggesting a saturation level consistent with Teklehaimanot et al. (2004). Similar to temperature the effect of rainfall is not directly related to the human infection, but rainfall influences the vector population abundance by providing surface water for breeding. A positive effect of rainfall on malaria transmission has been consistently reported in the literature; nevertheless, some studies have shown negative or neutral effects (Shililu et al. 1998, Lindsay et al. 2000b, Shanks et al. 2002, Singh and Sharma 2002, Abeku et al. 2003). This could be explained by the overwhelming effect of the temperature. For rainfall to have a positive effect in malaria infection, the temperature must be warm enough to support mosquitoes and parasite development (Bodker et al. 2003). This is supported by the low malaria transmission in the highland area where, rainfall is abundant but temperatures are below 20°C.

The individual effect of relative humidity on malaria infection, compared to temperature and rainfall, is less reported in the literature. We found that, average relative humidity of the previous month has a positive effect (higher than rainfall) on *P. falciparum* infection cases, in line with the findings by Bi et al. (2003). We were aware of the strong correlation between rainfall and relative humidity, therefore an interaction term was included in the model. We therefore believe that what is observed is the individual effect of relative humidity on *P. falciparum* infection risk. The humidity observed ranges from 15% to 80% with an average of 50% mainly driven by rainfall and temperature. We found that at a relative humidity below 60% there is a reduction of *P. falciparum* infection cases. This could be explained by reducing the vector lifespan in these conditions, reducing the proportion of survival (Pampana 1969). A minimum of 60% is required for the vector. In contrast, above 60% of relative humidity, the infection rate increases substantially with an increase of humidity. The risk at 80% is two times higher than the risk at 60%. This could be a result of better survival of the vector population.

The effect of the combined parameters (rainfall-humidity, temperature-humidity and temperature-rainfall) on *P. falciparum* infection incidence was small. This could be explained by the strong independent effects of each individual parameter.

In conclusion, our findings confirmed the strong association of weather on malaria infection. Although rainfall and relative humidity are important, temperature was the main driving force.

4.1.2.3 Effect of weather on mosquito dynamics (Objective 3) The mosquito population in this area is dominated by *Culex quinquefasciatus* species, largely present in the semi-urban site (Nouna). This is explained by *Culex* mosquitoes being able to breed in any kind of open-surface water, such as what is available in urban sites. The second largest population is the female *An. gambiae* species which is the main malaria vector. The vector distribution is similar to what was observed by Traoré (2003). The largest number of vectors throughout the year was caught in Goni, probably due the flooded rice cultivation activities creating a swampy area. In addition, there is a man-made lake in the village centre which is probably an additional source of mosquitoes. Contrary to our expectation in Kodougou, a rural site by a perennial river with traditional irrigated agricultural practices, we observed the lowest number of vectors. This could be explained by the rainfall condition, which was particularly low that year or else by insecticide to protect against the mosquitoes nuisance. Unfortunately this explanation could not be cross checked because of the failure of the rainfall sensor in this site. Mosquitoes sampling bias could be excluded as this finding was consistent for both HLC and LTC methods.

We observed a very high seasonal pattern of *An. gambiae* abundance. About 95% were caught during the rainy season (from June to October). Very few were caught during the dry season. This is explained by the rainfall providing breeding sites, reducing the temperature (about 28°C) and increasing the relative humidity (80%); thereby, creating optimal conditions for vector development. The dry season (November–May) is characterised by a total absence of rainfall and can be subdivided into cold and hot period. The cold period (November–January) follows the rainy season and in principle residual breeding sites from the rainy season should produce mosquitoes. However, the process is probably suppressed by the cold weather, known to slow down mosquito development. In contrast, in the hot period (February–April) temperatures are too high (40°C) leading to the clearance of breeding sites by evaporation and increased vector mortality. The few mosquitoes caught in this period probably resulted from breeding sites created around wells by water poured during the water-fetching process.

The key factor analysis done by estimating the *k-value* (vector generation log mortality) (Rogers 1983) shows a clear seasonal impact on the vector abundance. The *k-value* expresses the number of vectors that survived from the immature stage (egg) to the adult stage. The very high mortality observed in the dry season is explained by the absence of rainfall and the very hot and cold temperature. The sudden decrease of mortality in July (Figure 3.16) can be explained by the onset of the rainy season and the drop in temperature to levels suitable for vector survival. Surprisingly, there was increased vector mortality, consistently observed in all sites during the rainy season. This is probably attributable to the so-called density dependant mortality (Rogers 1983). This occurs when there is saturation of the environmental carrying capacity and individuals have to compete for limited resources and when there is increased presence of predator (Depinay et al. 2004). Despite the high mortality in this period and because of the high-level of abundance, there remained enough vectors to transmit the disease.

Because small number of *An. gambiae* caught during the dry season, the gravid rate calculated for months in this period could be highly biased. Therefore our focus will be on the rainy season. A high proportion of gravid (43%) vectors were caught in August consistently in all the four sites, suggesting a relatively old vector population. This could be the result of the onset of the rainy season in the previous months resulting in a significant decrease of mortality. Mosquitoes caught in August were therefore from July as the captures were performed in the first two weeks of the month. The significant decrease of the gravid population in following months, suggesting a much younger population, can be explained by the increased density-dependant mortality resulting in the death of old mosquitoes. Also breeding sites and the moderate temperature, allow the development of new mosquitoes. The parity rate, which was based on the unfed dissected mosquito from the rainy season showed some differences between the sites and month (August and September) as well. This population is the so-called "epidemiological dangerous population", because it represents the vectors which have oviposited at least once in their life, and therefore likely to be infectious. They also represent the old group of the vector population.

In conclusion, mosquito population dynamics are strictly weather dependant and highly seasonal in the study area. Most of vectors were caught during the rainy season. However vectors are also present in the dry season resulting in transmission throughout year. The mortality is very high in the dry season because of high temperature and absence of water and in the rainy season because of density dependent mortality.

4.1.2.4 Seasonal transmission pressure (Objective 4) The transmission pressure was assessed by calculating the biting rate and the EIR as in others studies (Onori and Grab 1980, Shiluli et al. 2003). In contrast to other studies that used sporozoite positive mosquitoes (Traoré 2003, Shiluli et al. 2004), we used parous mosquitoes as a proxy. We assumed that all parous mosquitoes captured were *anthropophagic* (feed exclusively on human). This assumption was based upon two reasons. First, previous studies in the same area showed a very small proportion of *zoophagic* vector among *An. Gambiae* (Traoré 2003). Similarly, Wanji et al. (2003) reported only less than 2% of non *anthropophagic* vectors in the mount Cameroon region. Second, the mosquitoes used were from the HLC methods, and it is unlikely that a *zoophagic* vector would land on a human for feeding. The results found by this approach are in good agreement with those which use the sporozoite methods. This method could be therefore a cost-effective alternative for assessing transmission pressure, since the sporozoite method is very demanding and needs ELISA facilities, which are not always affordable. Other aspects of transmission pressures were first assessed before the EIR. They are sporogony cycle, the VC and the biting rate.

As already defined the sporogonic cycle expressed the development of malaria parasites within the vector. The duration of this cycle is a key parameter in the vectorial capacity and the transmission pressure (Mcdonald 1957). The longer it takes, the lower the transmission pressure will be, as not enough vectors will live long enough to transmit the disease. This cycle was defined by Mcdonald 1957 to be strictly temperature dependent. Therefore, in a region with high seasonal climate variability it is inappropriate to estimate an average duration of the cycle. This was supported by our findings which showed monthly variation driven by the unstable temperature. Longer durations of the cycle observed in December and January in all the sites may be explained by the cold temperature at this period. In March and April the temperatures are particularly high, therefore the cycle is shorter (less than ten days).

We observed that *An. gambiae* vectors mostly bite late at night, in agreement with other studies (Charlwood et al. 2003, Wanji et al. 2003). Some vectors started biting early (by 18:00), when darkness sets in, however, the majority fed very late at night (21:00 to 04:00). This late biting suggested that most of the malaria transmission to children occurred indoors as children go to bed early. Due to the early beginning of feeding activities among a small proportion of vectors, children remain exposed to biting before going to bed, confirming that using a mosquito net cannot totally prevent exposure to mosquito bites. This was a concern raised regarding the negative effects of large-scale use of mosquito nets that may interact with the development of child immunity (Snow et al. 1998b). Another concern was the shifting of the vector feeding behaviour to early biting when the host is accessible (Magesa et al. 1991, Mbogo et al. 1996, Takken 2002). We cannot make any judgment about the hypothesis as the mosquito net use, though high (50%) due to an ongoing study was only among children and most adults remained unprotected. The study design was not set up to test this particular mosquito net hypothesis and this should be addressed in a separate study. The key message here is that, it is likely that transmission mainly occurred indoors, although one may argue that in this region there is a tendency of sleeping outside when indoor temperature is high. However, this outside sleeping phenomenon is only common during the hottest season, when the transmission is low.

VC developed by McDonald (1957), is an important indicator for the malaria transmission pressure. As we have observed in our findings, although it varies between sites, the seasonal pattern is consistent. We can see that the transmission in this area is perennial in line with the observed incidence of *P. falciparum* infection with seasonal peak. VC is driven by the vector abundance and temperature that affect the vector development and the biting frequency. The high VC observed during the rainy season is again the result of rainfall and moderate temperature. This has been also shown to be high during the rainy season by Lindsay et al. (1991). The particularly high VC in the Goni site is explained by the high number of vectors.

We estimated our biting rate and EIR based on an adult population assuming that it is similar to the children as it would have been unethical to use children. The number of infective bites a person received per night was highly seasonal and correlated with the vector abundance. As expected, the rainy season is the most dangerous period for mosquito biting in line with Traoré (2003). An annual average biting rate is less informative as there is high seasonal variation. The high variation between sites, suggests that a region wide biting rate is biased. We found the daily biting rate in Goni is about three times higher than the one in Nouna just 20km away. This highlights the importance of local assessment of malaria transmission risk. Similar findings were observed with the EIR (the infectious bite per night). Although we have used a proxy for calculating the EIR, the results agree with those of Traoré (2003). This suggests that our methods could be a cheaper alternative. We surprisingly observed a low biting rate and EIR in Kodougou. This result does not correlate with the observed incidence cases of *P. falciparum* infection which was high. This could be explained by the inverse relationship between high transmission pressure and malaria infection incidence. Indeed, it has been reported that people exposed to high EIR are likely to develop partial immunity faster and therefore become less susceptible to malaria, compared to those exposed to low EIR.

In conclusion we have demonstrated that malaria transmission pressure is driven by seasonal changes of the climate with the pressure being highest in the rainy season. We have also shown that transmission pressure can vary from one ecological setting to another at local scale, suggesting that microepidemiological studies are more appropriate to better understand transmission dynamics. Finally, we have shown that a simple and low cost approach can be used to assess transmission pressure. The EIR rather than being based on sporozoite detection (ELISA test) can simply be based on dissection to identify infectious vector (basis for the EIR calculation). Given all the above, are we able to predict *P. falciparum* infection?

4.1.3 Weather based predicting of P falciparum Infection at local scale (study question 2, objective 5)

We developed a dynamic model of malaria transmission among children under five. The model is composed of five difference equations expressing the changes in infection status of the human and vector population given temperature and rainfall conditions. The model simulated the vector population abundance and the human *P. falciparum* infection incidence for each of the three ecological settings over the year. Most of the model parameters were calculated based on the field data and fitted. The model is therefore driven by time series field data on vector, parasite and meteorological data, leading to a fair simulation of real-life malaria transmission dynamics. Both vector abundance and *P. falciparum* Incidence output of the model were in good agreement with the field observation.

4.1.3.1 Simulation of mosquito dynamics Vector population abundance is driven by rainfall and temperature. Our dynamic model represented this aspect in all the sites for which simulation was made. The peak vector abundance observed about two weeks after a peak of rainfall (Figure 3.21) is characteristic of the vector–rainfall relationship. Indeed, the development process of the vector from the egg to adult stage takes about 14 days in ideal temperature (28°C) conditions (Jepson et al. 1947, Depinay et al. 2004). The presence of water pools generated by rainwater allows the mosquitoes to lay their eggs which then develop into adult mosquitoes if the water pools are sustained for at least 14 days. Some potential breeding sites could be expected in the surrounding area of wells throughout the year. This is because of the constant pouring of water when people are fetching it. Usually an intentional pool is created for purposes of watering cattle. However, these pools are not common and only generate few mosquitoes. Because of the dry conditions of the area the most important source of breeding sites remains rainfall water and this explains the high abundance of mosquitoes in the rainy season. The presence of the perennial river in Kodougou did not impact on the mosquitoes abundances. This suggests that, as shown by our model prediction, rainfall is the main driver of the vector abundance. As expected in all sites the model detected few daily numbers of vectors (less that ten) during the dry season probably because of breeding sites created around wells.

The comparison of the monthly prediction to the number of vectors caught in the field showed, in general, a similar pattern for all the sites. This suggests the model is a good representation of the mosquito population dynamics. Some discrepancy in the timing of the peak abundance was observed in Cissé (Figure 3.22). There was a deviation of one month between the peak of the predicted number of vectors (September) and the observed one (August). This could bebecause of the soil texture in Cissé, which probably holds water less on the surface for a time long enough to allow vector development. This could not be captured by the model. Consistently in all sites the model detected some vectors in May and June though the field data showed no vectors. This could be explained by the fact the model is sensitive to any amount of rainfall. In the field, the quantity of rainfall observed in May and June was not enough to sustain vector breeding sites.

Although the model showed a fair representation of the mosquito population, it could be improved by also simulating the immature stage (eggs, larvae, pupae) of the vector which are strictly dependant on surface water availability. Mosquitoes need water to produce and the oviposition rate is assumed to be proportional to the mosquito number and the daily rainfall filling the water pools (Hoshen et al. 2004). Further, direct correlation of rainfall amount with mosquito abundance could result in some estimation bias. This is because water pool availability and duration is not only dependant on rainfall, but also on evaporation index, the soil texture and moisture index. High evaporation will cause quick-drying out of the pools, while a lower consistence of soil texture and dry soil will lead to fast infiltration.

4.1.3.2 Simulation of P. falciparum infection cases The good fit of the mathematical model output to the observed *P. falciparum* infection incidence suggests the model is indeed a good representation of the transmission dynamics (Figure 3.23). Although some monthly discrepancies were observed probably because of the small number of cases, the general seasonal pattern was well captured. The model is not sensitive to the sporogonic cycle. This means that small variations in ambient temperature, which is the principal driving factor of the cycle, will not result in major changes to the incidence level. Similarly, time from human infection to gametocyte development is not a key element in determining the incidence level.

The vector daily biting rate was found to be 0.56 per day. This would represent a gonotrophic cycle of 1.5 days if every bite achieves a full blood meal. However, this is not always the case, as often a mosquito will return for a second bite if it was interrupted. Thus, the gonotrophic cycle may be longer than found in this model. The model is insensitive to precise values of b, humans bitten per day and this reduces the validity of the model as an estimator of the gonotrophic cycle length. In addition, the model was developed assuming all vectors are *anthropophillic,* which is not necessarily the case. In fact, we expect this parameter to vary from one season to another (Awolola et al. 2002).

The incidence of malaria is highly dependent on two key parameters, which are the daily mortality rate of the vector and the parasite clearance rate in humans. These parameters can both be influenced by public health interventions. The daily mortality rate of the vector can be increased by vector control methods such as indoor residual spraying and vector number reduced by elimination of breeding sites. Effective treatment of patients will increase the malaria clearance rate in human (q) thus, protecting not only the sick individuals but also the surrounding population. The parasitological clearance rate (12%) is slightly slower than can be deduced from Müller et al. (2003) who found 27% seven days parasitological failure. This would reflect 17% daily clearance. This discrepancy is probably a result of Müller et al. (2003) measuring the asexual form clearance, while our focus was on the sexual form.

The model is driven by the parasitological data for children under five, while the entire population is contributing to the transmission process. To fully account for this effect we would need a survey of the general population. This would require checking large numbers of asymptomatic individuals for sub-clinical infections. This raised technical and ethical issues. Nevertheless, we assumed the under five parasite prevalence will not be unlike that of the general population.

In conclusion, the model has shown a potential for local scale seasonal prediction of *P. falciparum* infection. It could therefore be used to understand malaria transmission dynamics using meteorological parameters as the driving force. However we do not pretend to have captured 100% of the transmission dynamics. Further improvement could be made as the basic rule of a model as according to McKenzie (2000) is "A model is useful if it sharpens questions, points to what is missing in our data or in our conceptual grasp, and contributes to a larger process of discovery that will render it obsolete; a model that cannot be shown to be wrong is typically of little use" (McKenzie 2000, page 512).

4.1.4 Limitations

Although, we put maximum effort in the design and implementation of this study some limits were observed at different levels. These are limits inherent to any study and while they do not compromise the soundness of the results, in some case they make the interpretation of some results more difficult. These limits are summarised in Table 4.1. Possible solutions are proposed for future studies.

4.2 Conclusion

From our knowledge, this was the first attempt to model malaria transmission risk in Burkina Faso at a local scale. The major strength of this project was the comprehensive time series data, including community based infection data, vector data and weather data used to drive the dynamic model. Despite the workload on the data collection the fieldwork team and study participants, the surveys were successfully completed with a high participation rate.

We have demonstrated that *P. falciparum* infection incidence in all the four sites is perennial with high seasonal variation. The transmission peak is in the rainy season. Children in Goni and Kodougou have the highest incidence of *P. falciparum* infection. Nouna, a semi-urban site has the lowest *P. falciparum* infection. However, in multivariate model using conventional logistic regression, only children in Kodougou have shown significant increase of odds of *P. falciparum* infection compared to whose in Nouna. This difference was cancelled in a random effect model when we considered individual and household level variation. Suggesting that, at given same conditions (individual and household) the odds of *P. falciparum* infection are similar in all the sites.

P. falciparum infection among children is regulated by weather which impacts on the malaria vector dynamics. Although all the individual weather parameters (with a lag of one month) have an impact on *P. falciparum* infection, mean temperature is the best predictor and was the main driving force.

The mosquito population was mainly of the *Culex* species caught mainly in the semi-urban site (Nouna). Among the malaria vectors, *An. gambiae* is the most prominent specie. Its population dynamics are highly regulated by temperature and rainfall. Goni because of its ecological setting has the largest vector population.

The transmission pressure (EIR) is also highly seasonal and varies significantly and among sites. It was high in Goni, because of vector abundance. This has led to a high incidence of *P. falciparum* infection. Surprisingly, the transmission pressure was low in Kodougou despite its proximity to a perennial river.

We were finally able to develop and test a dynamic model of malaria transmission using the knowledge generated by this comprehensive time series

Table 4.1 Overview of the study limitations and possible impact and solutions

Level	Limitation	Possible impact	Solution
Infection data	Only febrile children were tested for *P. falciparum* infection	Underestimation of *P. falciparum* infection incidence as non-febrile child are possible carriers and contribute to the transmission dynamic	Test systematically all the children regardless of their febrile status
	Low sensitivity of Microscope test for *P. falciparum* detection	Possible underestimation of the *P. falciparum* infection incidence among febrile children. Only half of them tested positive	PCR (Polymerase Chain Reaction) for antibody. High sensitivity about 98 %. However, this method is only necessary for drug trials
Entomology data	Mosquitoes only caught on the 1st and 2nd days of the month assumed to be representative for the whole month.	Underestimation of the vector monthly abundance as there is a four-week gap between two captures which is enough time for new mosquitoes to grow and die before the next capture takes place	Perform captures every week or every two weeks or else capitalise on the LTC methods and perform a continuous capture over the study period
Entomology data	Human biting rate was calculated assuming all mosquitoes feed only on humans	Possible over estimation of the human biting rate as a small proportion may feed on animals	PCR test of mosquitoes for Human Blood Index
	EIR calculation was based on Parous mosquitoes	Possible over estimation of EIR	ELISA test of unfed mosquitoes for sporozoite detection
Weather data	The weather station for Goni site was located five Km away in Toni	Although the station was still within the recommended range, this could have introduced bias in the comparison with other sites	Weather data should be measured at the same site where infection survey and entomological survey are taking place
	The failure of the rainfall sensor in Kodougou	Kodougou was excluded in assessing weather impact on *P. falciparum* infection as well as in the dynamic model prediction. This reduced the statistical power	Acquire spare sensors at the beginning of the measurement. This will allow immediate replacement of any defective sensors thereby avoiding an interruption of measurement
Dynamic model level	The use of absolute rainfall	Assuming that the quantity of rainfall recorded is equal to what is available on the ground can be a source of bias as a portion is lost because of infiltration or evaporation	A water balance model to quantify the exact quantity of rain available on the ground

data and the results provided by the different analyses. The dynamic model driven by temperature and rainfall successfully simulated seasonal vector abundance for each site. It also predicted successfully the monthly malaria incidence. However, the model needs to be tested for longer periods as this year was not an average year for weather parameters.

We believe that though our study and results have some limitations, we can still make some recommendations.

4.2.1 Implications for public health

At this stage, it is probably premature to state the outputs of our study will have a public health impact. However, we have contributed to understand the complex relationship between malaria transmission and meteorological factors at local scale. The non-spatial model developed has demonstrated that some key factors are determinant for the sustainability of malaria transmission. Some of theses factors can be influenced by control strategies. These factors are malaria vector mortality and human parasite clearance, which when substantially increased can lead to reducing transmission. The first can be increased by a vector control program including indoor insecticide spray, systematic elimination of potential breeding site by drainage and larvicide spray. The second can be decreased by systematic detection and treatment with effective anti-malaria drugs. Since *P. falciparum* infection has been demonstrated to be low in the dry season, an intervention aimed at increasing the human parasite clearing will be more cost effective if undertaken in this period. This is motivated by the fact that in the dry season there will be few cases to treat. Also suppressing the parasite reservoir will lead to less infectious vectors during the rainy season.

This was the first attempt for systematic risk assessment of malaria based of meteorological factors using a dynamic model in Burkina Faso. Although, they are still some improvements needed we have paved the way for malaria modelling and systematic risk assessment. We therefore hope other researches will build on our work and come out with a model including additional aspects such as, space, health care systems, health care seeking behaviour, drug resistance, intervention programs and other important factors in malaria transmission. This will allow the model to be used as a tool to support intervention policy.

4.2.2 Lessons learned

- Malaria infection is highly seasonal and the pressure is high during the rainy season, however the infection is present throughout the year in the Kossi province.
- EIR estimation based on parous vectors can be a cost-effective alternative for evaluating malaria transmission pressure.
- A simple dynamic model of malaria risk at local scale is possible and can provide better insights into the transmission process. However it requires

well-defined and comprehensive time series data collection including infection, vector and weather data.

4.2.3 Recommendations for decisions makers

National level

- Malaria risk assessment is a prerequisite for a successful control programme since it is helpful for targeted intervention. In our study we have demonstrated that meteorological factors are strong predictors of malaria risk. We therefore suggest that, the Health Information Systems in Burkina Faso should integrate meteorological data generated by the National Meteorological Office. The data should be systematically analysed to assess the association with malaria and maybe other weather related diseases. If affordable, one digital weather station should be installed in each health district.
- Initiate a country-wide malaria transmission risk mapping research that can be regularly (every two years) updated with the support of Health Information Systems data, specific and localised studies and satellite data. This will have the double benefit of refining control programmes and evaluating their impact.

Health district level (Nouna)

- This study has demonstrated that although malaria transmission is clustered in the rainy season (from July to September), there is still some considerable transmission going on during the dry season. Therefore, prevention, detection and treatment efforts in the district should continue throughout the year.
- Given the high incidence observed in Goni and Kodougou, particular measures should be taken. This could include health education for reducing man-made vector breeding sites; prepare the referral health centres to cope with the increased number of malaria cases during the rainy season and implement active detection and treatment.
- The health district should make good use of the unique time series meteorological data provided by this project.

4.2.4 Recommendation for further research

Although malaria is a global problem, its transmission is driven by local conditions; therefore, understanding the transmission dynamics and reasons behind at this level, remains an important way to support control strategies. Garnham (1929) stated that "*the problem of malaria is so essentially a local one... that it makes the study of the disease a piece of research for every locality*". We therefore recommend that studies aiming to understand malaria transmission should first be local.

- Environmental factors have a great impact on the immature stage (larvae pupae) of malaria. This stage is highly important for the life cycle of the vector. We therefore suggest that future entomological studies in this region should map and characterise mosquito breeding to develop a local scale mosquito dynamic model including immature and adult stages.
- There is insufficient knowledge in the region regarding the malaria vector subspecies and their behaviour. Yet this is important for the development of effective malaria control programmes. We therefore suggest that future entomological studies should focus on identifying malaria vector subspecies (taxonomy) and their behaviours (biting, resting, flying distance, breeding preferences and others).
- Farming has been shown in this study and others as a risk factor for malaria infection. However there is a lack of studies in this region that systematically quantify the effect of land use, agriculture practice and malaria transmission. We therefore recommend a study that will fill this gap.
- We have demonstrated that rainfall is one of the key factors for the presence and development of the malaria vectors. However just using the amount of rainfall to assess malaria risk or vector abundance could be misleading. Future research should aim to develop a hydrological or water balance model to capture the precise amount of water available on the ground and the possible duration. This is helpful in modelling the immature stage of the vector and could improve our model.
- Ethnicity has been suggested to play a role in genetic susceptibility, the Fulani being less susceptible compared to others (Modiano et al. 1996, 1999). However our study did not confirm this. We therefore suggest a study in this Nouna area to see whether Fulani are less susceptible to malaria compared to others if all other factors are considered. If yes is it attributable to genetic factors or to their nomadic lifestyle?

4.2.5 Next steps

The overall project was designed to develop a comprehensive malaria transmission model that included both non-spatial and spatial models as extensively discussed in the introduction chapter. The first was to be used for point and temporal prediction of *P. falciparum* infection in villages where malaria and entomological survey could not take place, using weather data provided by satellite. The second could have used the point and temporal prediction to build an area wide malaria risk model resulting in risk maps.

The non-spatial model was developed and successfully tested as shown in this dissertation. However, a spatial model is still needed for area wide prediction with the support of climate models, land use model and remote sensing data. The next step will therefore be the development of such a model. All necessary data including ground and remote sensing data are now available. The analysis and results will be presented in our next book. This work has therefore paved the ground for the next step in developing a high resolution spatial model for malaria transmission in the Kossi province and for further studies aiming to assess the risk of malaria transmission.

To allow the non-spatial model to be used for prediction, we have planned to develop a computer program with a user-friendly interface. This interface will allow the input of temperature and rainfall data and modification of some of the model parameters. Given these inputs, the programs will calculate the number of *P. falciparum* infection monthly for 12 months for a given location. This computer program will be designed for the health district level and will be presented in our next edition.

References

Abeku TA, van Oortmarssen GJ, Borsboom G, de Vlas SJ, Habbema JD. (2003) Spatial and temporal variations of malaria epidemic risk in Ethiopia: factors involved and implications. *Acta Trop* 87:331–40.

Anderson RM and May RM. (1991). *Infectious Disease of Humans. Dynamics and Control*. Oxford University Press, UK.

Ansari MA, Razdan RK. (2004) Impact of residual spraying of Reldan against Anopheles culicifacies in selected villages of District Ghaziabad (Uttar Pradesh), *India. J Vector Borne Dis* 41:54–60.

Ansell J, Hamilton KA, Pinder M, Walraven GE, Lindsay SW. (2002) Short-range attractiveness of pregnant women to Anopheles gambiae mosquitoes. *Trans R Soc Trop Med Hyg* 96:113–6.

Aronoff S. (1989) *Geographical Information Systems: A Management Perspective*. WDL Publication, Ottawa.

Awolola TS, Okwa, Hunt RH, Ogunrinade AF, Coetzee M. (2002) Dynamics of the malaria vector populations in coastal Lagos, south-western Nigeria. *Ann. Trop.Med Parasitol* 96:75–82.

Baldet T, Diabate A, Guiguemde TR. (2003) Malaria transmission in 1999 in the rice field area of the Kou Valley (Bama), (Burkina Faso) *Santé* 13:55–60.

Becher H. (2004) General Principles of Data Analysis: Continuous covariables in epidemiological studies. In: Ahrens W, Pigeot I, editors. *Handbook of Epidemiology*. Heidelberg: Springer, pp:611–612.

Beier JC, Killeen GF, Githure JI. (1999) Short report: entomologic inoculation rates and P. falciparum malaria prevalence in Africa. *Am J Trop Med Hyg*. 61:109–13.

Beier JC, Oster CN, Onyango FK, Bales JD, Sherwood JA, Perkins PV, Chumo DK, Koech DV, Whitmire RE, Roberts CR, et al. (1994) P. falciparum incidence relative to entomologic inoculation rates at a site proposed for testing malaria vaccines in western Kenya. *Am J Trop Med Hyg* 50:529–36.

Bi P, Tong S, Donald K, Parton KA, Ni J. (2003) Climatic variables and transmission of malaria: a 12-year data analysis in Shuchen County, China. *Public Health Rep* 118:65–71.

Biritwum RB, Welbeck J, Barnish G. (2000) Incidence and management of malaria in two communities of different socio-economic level, in Accra, Ghana. *Ann Trop Med Parasitol* 94:771–8.

Bodker R, Akida J, Shayo D, Kisinza W, Msangeni HA, Pedersen EM, Lindsay SW. (2003) Relationship between altitude and intensity of malaria transmission in the Usambara Mountains, Tanzania. *J Med Entomol* 40:706–17.

Booman M, Durrheim DN, La Grange K, Martin C, Mabuza AM, Zitha A, Mbokazi FM, Fraser C, Sharp BL. (2000) Using a geographical information system to plan a malaria control programme in South Africa. *Bull World Health Organ* 78:1438–44.

Bradley DJ, Newbold CI, and Warrell DA. (1987) Malaria. In: *Oxford Textbook of Medicine*. Eds: Weatherall DJ, Ledingham JGG, and Warrell DA. Oxford University Press, Oxford.

Bremen J. (2001) The ears of the hippopotamus: manifestations, determinants, and estimates of the malaria burden. *Am J Trop Med Hyg* 64: 1–11.

Brêtas G. (1995) Geographical Information System for the study and control of in GIS for Health and Environment: Proceedings of an International Workshop held in Colombo, Sri Lanka, 5–10 September 1994, IDRC ISBN 0-88936-766–3.

Bryce J, Boschi-Pinto C, Shibuya K, Black RE. (2005) WHO estimates of the causes of death in children, *Lancet* 365: 1147–52.

Burrough PA and McDonnell PA. (1998) *Principles of Geographical Information Systems*. Oxford University Press, Oxford.

Carter R, Mendis KN, Roberts D. (2000) Spatial targeting of interventions against malaria. *Bull World Health Organ* 78:1401–11.

Charlwood JD, Pinto J, Ferrara PR, Sousa CA, Ferreira C, Gil V, Do Rosario VE. (2003) Raised houses reduce mosquito bites. *Malar J* 2:45.

Charlwood JD, Qassim M, Elnsur EI, Donnelly M, Petrarca V, Billingsley PF, Pinto J, Smith T. (2001) The impact of indoor residual spraying with Malathion on malaria in refugee camps in eastern Sudan. *Acta Trop* 80:1–8.

Clements AN. (1999) *The Biology of Mosquitoes – Volume 2 Sensory Reception and Behaviour* CABI Publishing, Wallingford.

Cot M, Brutus L, Pinell V, Ramaroson H, Raveloson A, Rabeson D, Rakotonjanabelo AL. (2002) Malaria prevention during pregnancy in unstable transmission areas: the highlands of Madagascar. *Trop Med Int Health* 7:565–72.

Craig MH, Snow RW, le Sueur D. (1999) A climate-based distribution model of malaria transmission in sub-Saharan Africa. *Parasitol Today* 15:105–11.

Craig MH, Kleinschmidt I, Nawn JB, Le Sueur D, Sharp BL. (2004) Exploring 30 years of malaria case data in KwaZulu-Natal, South Africa: Part I. The impact of climatic factors. *Trop Med Int Health* 9:1247–57.

DeMers MN. (1997) *Fundamentals of Geographical Information Systems*. New York: John Wiley and Son.

Depinay JM, Mbogo CM, Killeen G, Knols B, Beier J, Carlson J, Dushoff J, Billingsley P, Mwambi H, Githure J, Toure AM, McKenzie FE. (2004) A simulation model of African Anopheles ecology and population dynamics for the analysis of malaria transmission. *Malar J* 3:29.

Detinova TS. (1962) Age-grouping methods in Diptera of medical importance with special reference to some vectors of malaria. Monogr Ser WHO N° 47, Geneva.

Detinova TS. (1963) *Méthodes à appliquer pour classer par groupes d'âge les diptères présentant une importance médicale.* Ser Monogr WHO N°27, Geneva.

Dicko A, Mantel C, Kouriba B, Sagara I, Thera MA, Doumbia S, Diallo M, Poudiougou B, Diakite M, Doumbo OK. (2005) Season, fever prevalence and pyrogenic threshold for malaria disease definition in an endemic area of Mali. *Trop Med Int Health* 10:550–6.

Dietz K (1988) Density-dependence in parasite transmission dynamics. *Parasitol Today* 4:91–7.

Dietz K, Heesterbeek JAP. (2002) Daniel Bernoulli's epidemiological model revisited. *Math Bio Sci* 180:1–21.

Dietz K, Molineaux L, Thomas A. (1974) Malaria model tested in the savannah. *Bull World Health Organ* 50: 347–357.

Doke PP, Sathe RS, Chouhan SP, Bhosale AS. (2000) Impact of single round of indoor residual spray with lambda-cyhalotrin 10% WP on P. falciparum infection in Akola district, Maharashtra State. *J Commun Dis* 32:190–200.

Eisele TP, Keating J, Swalm C, Mbogo CM, Githeko AK, Regens JL, Githure JI, Andrews L, Beier JC. (2003) Linking field-based ecological data with remotely sensed data using a geographic information system in two malaria endemic urban areas of Kenya. *Malar J* 2:44.

Ettling MB, Shepard DS. (1991) Economic cost of malaria in Rwanda. *Trop Med Parasitol* 42: 214–8.

Gallup J. and Sachs J. (2001) The economic burden of malaria. *Am. J. Trop. Med. Hyg* 64: 85–96.

Gamage-Mendis AC, Carter R, Mendis C, De Zoysa AP, Herath PR, Mendis KN. (1991) Clustering of malaria infections within an endemic population: Risk of malaria associated with type of house construction. *Am J Trop Med Hyg* 45: 77–85.

Garrett-Jones C. (1964) The human blood index of malaria vectors in relation to epidemiological assessment. *Bull World Health Organ* 30:241–61.

Garnham PCC. (1929) Malaria in Kisumu, Kenya colony. *Journal of Tropical Medicine and Hygiene* 32:207–216.

Ghebreyesus TA, Haile M, Witten KH, Getachew A, Yohannes AM, Yohannes M, Teklehaimanot HD, Lindsay SW, Byass P. (1999) Incidence of malaria among children living near dams in northern Ethiopia: community based incidence survey. *BMJ* 319:663–6.

Ghebreyesus TA, Haile M, Witten KH, Getachew A, Yohannes M, Lindsay SW, Byass P. (2000) Household risk factors for malaria among children in the Ethiopian highlands. *Trans R Soc Trop Med Hyg* 94: 17–21.

Gill CA. (1920) The relationship between malaria and rainfall. *Indian Journal of Medical Research* 37: 618–632.

Gilles HM, Warrell DA. (1993) *Bruce-Chwatt's Essential Malariology,* Third edition. Edward Arnold, London.

Gillies MT and Coetzee M. (1987) *A supplement to the anopheline of Africa south of the Sahara*. Publications of South African Institute for Medical Research N° 55, Johannesburg.

Githeko, AK and Ndegwa W. (2001) Predicting malaria epidemics in Kenyan highlands using climate data: a tool for decision makers. *Glob Change Hum Health* 2:54–63.

Goldstein H, Rasbash J. (1996) Improved approximations for multilevel models with binary responses. *J Roy Stat Soc* 159:505–13.

Greenland S. (2000) Principles of multilevel modeling. *Int J Epidemiol* 29:158–67.

Gu W, Killeen GF, Mbongo CM, Regens JL, Githure JI, Beier JC. (2003) An individual-based model of P. falciparum malaria transmission on the coast of Kenya. *Trans R Soc Trop Med Hyg* 97: 43–50.

Gunasekaran K, Sahu SS, Jambulingam P, Das PK. (2005) DDT indoor residual spray, still an effective tool to control Anopheles fluviatilis-transmitted P. falciparum malaria in India. *Trop Med Int Health* 10:160–8.

Haddow AJ. (1942) The mosquito fauna and climate of native hats at Kisumu, Kenya. *Bulletin of Entomological Research* 33:91–142.

Halloran ME, Struchiner CJ, Spielman A. (1989) Modellingmalaria vaccines. II: Population effects of stage-specific malaria vaccines dependent on natural boosting. *Math Biosci* 94: 115–149.

Hassan AN, Kenawy MA, Kamal H, Abdel Sattar AA, Sowilem MM. (2003) GIS-based prediction of malaria risk in Egypt. *East Mediterr Health J* 9:548–58.

Hawley WA, Phillips-Howard PA, ter Kuile FO, Terlouw DJ, Vulule JM, Ombok M, Nahlen BL, Gimnig JE, Kariuki SK, Kolczak MS, Hightower AW. (2003) Community-wide effects of permethrin-treated bed nets on child mortality and malaria morbidity in western Kenya. *Am J Trop Med Hyg* 68:121–7.

Hay SI, Omumbo JA, Craig MH and Snow RW. (2000) *Earth Observation, Geographic Information Systems and P. falciparum Malaria in Sub-Saharan Africa, Remote Sensing and Geographical Information System in Epidemiology*, Volume 47 Oxford, UK, pp 173–215.

Hay SI, Rogers DJ, Randolph SE, Stern DI, Cox J, Shanks GD, Snow RW. (2002) Hot topic or hot air? Climate change and malaria resurgence in East African highlands. *Trends Parasitol* 18:530–4.

Hay SI, Snow RW, Rogers DJ. (1998) Predicting malaria seasons in Kenya using multitemporal meteorological satellite sensor data. *Trans R Soc Trop Med Hyg* 92:12–20.

Himeidan YE, Elbashir MI, Adam I. (2004) Attractiveness of pregnant women to the malaria vector, Anopheles arabiensis, in Sudan. *Ann Trop Med Parasitol* 98:631.

Hoshen MB, Morse AP. (2004) A weather-driven model of malaria transmission. *Malaria J.* 3:32.

Jepson WF, Moutia A, Courtois C. (1947) The malaria problem in Mauritius: The binomics of Mauritian anophelines. *Bull Entomol Res* 38:177–208.

Kermack WO, McKendrick AG. (1927) Contributions to the mathematical theory of epidemics (Part I). *Proc Roy Soc Lond A* 115:700–721.

Kitron U, Pener H, Costin C, Orshan L, Greenberg Z, Shalom U. (1994) Geographic information system in malaria surveillance: mosquito breeding and imported cases in Israel. *Am J Trop Med Hyg* 50:550–6.

Kleinschmidt I, Bagayoko M, Clarke GP, Craig M, Le Sueur D. (2000) A spatial statistical approach to malaria mapping. *Int J Epidemiol* 29:355–61.

Kleinschmidt I, Sharp BL, Clarke GP, Curtis B, Fraser C. (2001a) Use of generalized linear mixed models in the spatial analysis of small-area malaria incidence rates in Kwazulu Natal, South Africa. *Am J Epidemiol* 153:1213–21.

Kleinschmidt I, Omumbo J, Briet O, van de Giesen N, Sogoba N, Mensah NK, Windmeijer P, Moussa M, Teuscher T. (2001b) An empirical malaria distribution map for West Africa. *Trop Med Int Health* 6:779–86.

Konradsen F, Amerasingle P, Van der Hoeck W, Amerasingle F, Per D, Piyaratne M. (2003) Strong association between house characteristic and malaria vectors in Sri Lanka. *Am J Trop Med Hyg* 68: 177–81.

Koudou BG, Tano Y, Doumbia M, Nsanzabana C, Cissé G, Girardin O, Dao D, N'Goran EK, Vounatsou P, Bordmann G, Keiser J, Tanner M, Utzinger J. (2005) Malaria transmission dynamics in central Cote d'Ivoire: the influence of changing patterns of irrigated rice agriculture. *Med Vet Entomol* 19:27–37.

Kovats RS, Campbell-Lendrum DH, McMichael AJ, Woodward A, Cox JS. (2001) Early effects of climate change: do they include changes in vector-borne disease? *Philos Trans R Soc Lond B Biol Sci* 356:1057–1068.

Le Sueur D, Binka F, Lengeler C, De Savigny D, Snow B, Teuscher T, Toure Y. (1997) An atlas of malaria in Africa. *Afr Health* 19:23–4.

Lengeler C. (2004) Insecticide treated bednets and curtains for preventing malaria. In: *The Cochrane Library*, Issue 2.

Lepes T. (1974) Present status of the global malaria eradication programme and prospects for the future. *J Trop Med Hyg* 77:47–53.

Lillesand TM and Kiefer RW. (1994) *Remote Sensing and Image Interpretation.* John Wiley & Sons, New York.

Lindblade KA, Walker ED, Onapa AW, Katungu J, Wilson ML. (1999) Highland malaria in Uganda: prospective analysis of an epidemic associated with El Nino. *Trans R Soc Trop Med Hyg* 93:480–7.

Lindblade KA, Walker ED, Onapa AW, Katungu J, Wilson ML. (2000) Land use change alters malaria transmission parameters by modifying temperature in a highland area of Uganda. *Trop Med Int Health* 5:263–74.

Lindsay SW, Wilkins HA, Zieler HA, Daly RJ, Petrarca V, Byass P. (1991) Ability of Anopheles gambiae mosquitoes to transmit malaria during the dry and wet seasons in an area of irrigated rice cultivation in The Gambia. *J Trop Med Hyg* 94:313–24.

Lindsay SW, Armstrong Schellenberg JR, Zeiler HA, Daly RJ, Salum FM, Wilkins HA. (1995) Exposure of Gambian children to Anopheles gambiae malaria vectors in an irrigated rice production area. *Med Vet Entomol* 9:50–8.

Lindsay SW, Birley MH. (1996) Climate change and malaria transmission. *Ann Trop Med Parasitol* 90:573–88.

Lindsay SW, Martens WJ. (1998) Malaria in the African highlands: past, present and future. *Bull World Health Organ* 76:33–45.

Lindsay SW, Ansell J, Selman C, Cox V, Hamilton K, Walraven G. (2000a) Effect of pregnancy on exposure to malaria mosquitoes. *Lancet* 355:1972.

Lindsay SW, Bodker R, Malima R, Msangeni HA, Kisinza W. (2000b) Effect of 1997–98 El Nino on highland malaria in Tanzania. *Lancet* 355:989–990.

Lindsay SW, Emerson PM, Charlwood JD. (2002) Reducing malaria by mosquito-proofing houses. *Trends Parasitol* 18: 510–4.

Lindsay SW, Jawara M, Paine K, Pinder M, Walraven GEL, Emerson PM. (2003) Changes in house design reduce exposure to malaria mosquieos. *Trop Med Int Health* 8: 512–517.

Loslier L. (1995) Geographical Information Systems (GIS) from health perspectives in GIS for Health and Environment: Proceedings of an International Workshop held in Colombo, Sri Lanka, 5–10 September 1994, IDRC ISBN 0-88936-766-3.

Luckner D, Lell B, Greve B, Lehman LG, Schmidt-Ott RJ, Matousek P, Herbich K, Schmid D, Mba R, Kremsner PG. (1998) No influence of socioeconomic factors on severe malarial anaemia, hyperparasitaemia or reinfection. *Trans R Soc Trop Med Hyg* 92:478–81.

Lusingu JP, Vestergaard LS, Mmbando BP, Drakeley CJ, Jones C, Akida J, Savaeli ZX, Kitua AY, Lemnge MM, Theander TG. (2004) Malaria morbidity and immunity among residents of villages with different P. falciparum transmission intensity in North-Eastern Tanzania. *Malar J* 3:26.

Lyimo EO, Takken W. (1993) Effect of body size on fecundity and pre gravid rate of Anopheles gambiae females in Tanzania. *Med Vet Entomol* 7:328–332.

Macdonald G. (1957) Appendix I. Mathematical statement. In: *The Epidemiology and Control of Malaria.* pp 201, Oxford University Press; London.

Macdonald G. (1968) The dynamics of malaria. *Bull World Health Organ* 38: 743–755.

Magesa SM, Wilkes TJ, Mnzava AE, Njunwa KJ, Myamba J, Kivuyo MD, Hill N, Lines JD, Curtis CF. (1991) Trial of pyrethroid impregnated bednets in an area of Tanzania holoendemic for malaria. Part 2. Effects on the malaria vector population. *Acta Trop* 49:97–108.

Malakooti MA, Biomndo K, Shanks GD. (1998) Reemergence of epidemic malaria in the highlands of western Kenya. *Emerg Infect Dis* 4:671–6.

MARA/ARMA. (1998) Towards an Atlas of Malaria Risk in Africa. First Technical Reports of the MARA/ARMA collaboration, Durban.

Marimbu J, Ndayiragije A, Le Bras M, Chaperon J. (1993) Environnement et paludisme au Burundi: A propos d'une epidemie de paludisme dans une region montagneuse non endemique. *Bull Soc Pathol Exot.* 86: 399–401.

Martens WJ, Niessen LW, Rotmans J, Jetten TH, McMichael AJ. (1995) Potential impact of global climate change on malaria risk. *Environ Health Perspect* 103:458–64.

Martens WJM. (1997) Health Impacts of climate Change and Ozone Depletion: En Eco-Epidemiological Modelling Approach. Doctoral thesis, Maastricht University.

Mauny F, Viel JF, Handschumacher P, Sellin B.(2004). Multilevel modelling and malaria: a new method for an old disease. *Int J Epidemiol* 33:1337–44.

May J, Horstmann R. (2004) Einfluss genetischer Varianten des Menschen uaf Resitenz und Immunität gegen Malaria. *Bundesgesundheitsbl-Gesundheitsforch-Gesundheitsschutz* 47:1000–1008.

Mbogo CN, Baya NM, Ofulla AV, Githure JI, Snow RW. (1996) The impact of permethrin-impregnated bednets on malaria vectors of the Kenyan coast. *Med Vet Entomol* 10:251–9.

Mbogo CN, Glass GE, Forster D, Kabiru EW, Githure JI, Ouma JH, Beier JC (1993). Evaluation of light traps for sampling anophlelin mosquitoes in kilifi, Kenya. *J Am Mosq Control Assoc* 9:260–3.

McKenzie FE. (2000) Why model malaria? *Parasitol Today* 16: 511–516.

McKenzie FE, Baird JK, Beier JC, Lal AA, Bossert WH. (2002) A biologic basis for integrated malaria control. *Am J Trop Med Hyg* 67: 571–577.

McKenzie FE, Samba EM. (2004) The role of mathematical modelling in evidence-based malaria control. *Am J Trop Med Hyg* 71:94–6.

Mills A. (1993) The household costs of malaria in Nepal. *Trop Med Parasitol* 44:9–13.

Minakawa N, Sonye G, Mogi M, Githeko A, Yan G. (2002) The effects of climatic factors on the distribution and abundance of malaria vectors in Kenya. *J Med Entomol* 39:833–41.

Ministére de la Santé (2001), *Annuaire statitique 2001*, Ouagadougou.

Modiano D, Petrarca V, Sirima BS, Nebie I, Diallo D, Esposito F, Coluzzi M. (1996) Different response to P. falciparum malaria in west African sympatric ethnic groups. *Proc Natl Acad Sci USA* 93:13206–11.

Modiano D, Sirima BS, Sawadogo A, Sanou I, Pare J, Konate A, Pagnoni F. (1998) Severe malaria in Burkina Faso: influence of age and transmission level on clinical presentation. *Am J Trop Med Hyg* 59: 539–542.

Modiano D, Chiucchiuini A, Petrarca V, Sirima BS, Luoni G, Roggero MA, Corradin G, Coluzzi M, Esposito F. (1999) Interethnic differences in the humoral response to non-repetitive regions of the P. falciparum circumsporozoite protein. *Am J Trop Med Hyg* 61:663–7.

Molineaux L and Gramiccia G (1980). *The Garki Project*. World Health Organization, Geneva. p. 311.

Müller O and Garenne M. (1999) Childhood mortality in sub-Saharan Africa. *Lancet* 353: 673.

Müller O.(2000) History of and state of Global malaria Control, *Nova Acta Leopoldina* 80: 127–149.

Müller O, Becher H, van Zweeden AB, Ye Y, Diallo DA, Konate AT, Gbangou A, Kouyate B, Garenne M. (2001) Effect of Zinc supplementation on P. falciparum malaria among African Children: A Randomized Controlled Trial. *BMJ* 322: 1567.

Müller O, Traoré C, Becher H, Kouyate B. (2003) Malaria morbidity, treatment-seeking behaviour, and mortality in a cohort of young children in rural Burkina Faso. *Trop Med Int Health* 8: 290–296.

Najera JA. (1989) Malaria and the work of WHO. *Bull World Health Organ* 67:229–43.

Nihei N, Hashida Y, Kobayashi M, Ishii A. (2002) Analysis of malaria endemic areas on the Indochina Peninsula using remote sensing. *Jpn J Infect Dis* 55:160–6.

Oaks SC, Mitchell VS, Pearson GW, Carpenter CCJ. (1991) *Malaria: obstacles and opportunities. A Report of the Institute of Medicine*, National Academy Press, Washington, D.C.

Okech BA, Gouagna LC, Walczak E, Kabiru EW, Beier JC, Yan G, Githure JI. (2004) The development of P. falciparum in experimentally infected Anopheles gambiae (Diptera: Culicidae) under ambient microhabitat temperature in western Kenya. *Acta Trop* 92:99–108.

Okoko BJ, Enwere G, Ota MO. (2003) The epidemiology and consequences of maternal malaria: a review of immunological basis. *Acta Trop* 87:193–205.

Omumbo JA, Ouma J, Rapuoda B, Craig MH, le Sueur D, Snow RW. (1998) Mapping malaria transmission intensity using geographical information systems (GIS): an example from Kenya. *Ann Trop Med Parasitol* 92:7–21.

Omumbo JA, Guerra CA, Hay SI, Snow RW. (2005) The influence of urbanisation on measures of P. falciparum infection prevalence in East Africa. *Acta Trop* 93:11–21.

Onori E, Grab B. (1980) Indicators for the forecasting of malaria epidemics. *Bull World Health Organ* 58:91–8.

Onori E, Beales P and Gilles H. (1993) From malaria eradication to malaria control: the past, the present and the future. In Gilles, H., and Warrel, D. (eds) *Bruce-Chwatt's Essential Malariology*; pp. 267–282.

Over M. (1993) The consequences of adult ill-health. In: Feachem, R., Kjoellstrom, T., Murray, C, Over, M, and Phillips M. (eds) (1993b): *Bruce-Chwatt's Essential Malariology*; pp. 196–226. Boston: Little, Brown and Company 1993b.

Palsson K, Jaenson TG, Dias F, Laugen AT, Bjorkman A. (2004) Endophilic Anopheles mosquitoes in Guinea Bissau, West Africa, in relation to human housing conditions. *J Med Entomol* 41:746–52.

Pampana E. (1969) *A Textbook of Malaria Eradication*. London: Oxford University Press.

Patz JA, Strzepek K, Lele S, Hedden M, Greene S, Noden B, Hay SI, Kalkstein L, Beier JC. (1998) Predicting key malaria transmission factors, biting and entomological inoculation rates, using modeled soil moisture in Kenya. *Trop Med Int Health* 3:818–27.

Patz JA. (2002) A human disease indicator for the effects of recent global climate change. *Proc Natl Acad Sci USA* 99: 12506–12508.

Piebe de Vries and Martens P. (2000) A CAMERA focus on Local Eco-epidemiological Malaria Risk Assessment, a model in development. Working paper 100-E001, Universiteit Maastricht ICIC. Maastricht.

Randolph SE, Rogers DJ. (2000) Satellite data and disease transmission by vectors: the creation of maps for risk prediction. *Bull Soc Pathol Exot* 93:207.

Rasbash J, Steele F, Brown W, Prosser B. (2004) *A User's Guide to MLwinN*, version 2.0. Centre for Multilevel Modelling, Institute of Education, University of London.

Reyburn H, Mbatia R, Drakeley C, Bruce J, Carneiro I, Olomi R, Cox J, Nkya WM, Lemnge M, Greenwood BM, Riley EM. (2005) Association of transmission intensity and age with clinical manifestations and case fatality of severe P. falciparum malaria. *JAMA* 293:1461–70.

Rogers DJ (1983) In Youdeowei A and Service MW, *Pest and Vector Management in the Tropics with Particular Reference to Insects, Ticks, Mites and Snails*. 1983, London: Longman, pp 139–159.

Rogers DJ, Randolph SE, Snow RW, Hay SI. (2002) Satellite imagery in the study and forecast of malaria. *Nature*. 415:710–5.

Ross R. (1911) *The Prevention of Malaria*. London: John Murray.

Ross R. (1928) *Studies on Malaria*. London: John Murray.

Royston P. (2000) A strategy for modelling the effects of continuous covariates in medicine and epidemiology. *Stat Med* 19:1831–1847.

Ruwende C, Khoo SC, Snow RW, Yates SN, Kwiatkowski D, Gupta S, Warn P, Allsopp CE, Gilbert SC, Peschu N et al. (1995) Natural selection of hemi- and heterozygotes for G6PD deficiency in Africa by resistance to severe malaria. *Nature* 376:246–9.

Sachs J and Malaney P. (2002) The economic and social burden of malaria. *Nature* 415:680–685.

Sauerborn R, Shepard DS, Ettling MB, Brinkmann U, Nougtara A, Diesfeld HJ. (1991) Estimating the direct and indirect economic costs of malaria in a rural district of Burkina Faso. *Trop Med Parasitol* 42:219–23.

Sauerborn R, Nougtara A, Hein M, Diesfeld HJ. (1996) Seasonal variations of the household costs of illness in Burkina Faso. *Soc. Sci. Med* 43: 281–90.

Sauerborn R and Karam M. (2000) Geographical Information Systems. In Lippeveld T, Sauerborn R, Bodart C. *Design and implementation of Health Information Systems*. WHO Monograph, Geneva, pp 213–224.

Schellenberg JA, Newell JN, Snow RW, Mung'ala V, Marsh K, Smith PG, Hayes RJ. (1998) An analysis of the geographical distribution of severe malaria in children in Kilifi District, *Kenya. Int J Epidemiol* 27:323–329.

Service MW. (1973) Identification of predators of Anopheles gambiae resting in huts, by the precipitin test. *Trans R Soc Trop Med Hyg* 67:33–34.

Shanks GD, Biomndo K, Hay SI, Snow RW. (2000) Changing patterns of clinical malaria since 1965 among a tea estate population located in the Kenyan highlands. *Trans R Soc Trop Med Hyg* 94:253–5.

Shanks GD, Hay SI, Stern DI, Biomndo K, Snow RW. (2002) Meteorologic influences on P. falciparum malaria in the Highland Tea Estates of Kericho, Western Kenya. *Emerg Infect Dis* 8:1404–8.

Shanks GD, Biomndo K, Guyatt HL, Snow RW. (2005) Travel as a risk factor for uncomplicated P. falciparum malaria in the highlands of western Kenya. *Trans R Soc Trop Med Hyg* 99:71–4.

Sharma VP and Sharma RC. (1989) Community based bio-environmental control of malaria in Kheda District, Gujarat, India. *J Am Mosq Control Assoc* 5: 514–521.

Sharma VP, Srivastava A, Nagpal BN. (1994) A study of the relationship of rice cultivation and annual parasite incidence of malaria in India. *Soc Sci Med* 38:165–78.

Sharma VP, Dhiman RC, Ansari, MA, Nagpal BN, Srivastava A, Kmanavalan P, Adiga S, Radhakrishinan K, Chandrasekhar MG. (1996) Study on the feasibility of delineating mosquito genic conditions in and around Delhi using India Remote Sensing Satellite data. *Indian J Malariol* 33: 107–125.

Sharma VP and Srivastava A. (1997) Role of geographic information systems in malaria control. *Indian J Malariol* 106: 198–204.

Shililu JI, Maier WA, Seitz H.M, Orago AS. (1998) Seasonal density, sporozoite rates and entomological inoculation rates of Anopheles gambiae and Anopheles funestus in a high-altitude sugarcane-growing zone in Western Kenya. *Trop Med Int Health* 3:706–10.

Shililu J, Ghebremeskel T, Mengistu S, Fekadu H, Zerom M, Mbogo C, Githure J, Novak R, Brantly E, Beier JC. (2003) High seasonal variation in entomologic inoculation rates in Eritrea, a semi-arid region of unstable malaria in Africa. *Am J Trop Med Hyg* 69:607–13.

Shililu J, Ghebremeskel T, Seulu F, Mengistu S, Fekadu H, Zerom M, Asmelash GE, Sintasath D, Mbogo C, Githure J, Brantly E, Beier JC, Novak RJ. (2004) Seasonal abundance, vector behavior, and malaria parasite transmission in Eritrea. *J Am Mosq Control Assoc* 20:155–64.

Singh N, Singh OP, Sharma VP. (1996) Dynamics of malaria transmission in forested and deforested regions of Mandla District, central India. *J Am Mosq Control Assoc* 12:225–234.

Singh N, Sharma VP. (2002) Patterns of rainfall and malaria in Madhya Pradesh, central India. *Ann Trop Med Parasitol* 96: 349–59.

Sissoko MS, Dicko A, Briet OJ, Sissoko M, Sagara I, Keita HD, Sogoba M, Rogier C, Toure YT, Doumbo OK. (2004) Malaria incidence in relation to rice cultivation in the irrigated Sahel of Mali. *Acta Trop* 89:161–70.

Smith TA, Leuenberger R, Lengeler C. (2001) Child mortality and malaria transmission intensity in Africa. *Trends Parasitol.* 17:145–9.

Snow J. (1855) *On the Mode of Communication of Cholera.* London, Churchill (Reprinted in Snow on cholera: a reprint of two papers. New York, Hafner Publishing company, 1965).

Snow RW, Omumbo JA, Lowe B, Molyneux CS, Obiero JO, Palmer A, Weber MW, Pinder M, Nahlen B, Obonyo C, Newbold C, Gupta S, Marsh K. (1997) Relation between severe malaria morbidity in children and level of P. falciparum transmission in Africa. *Lancet* 349: 1650–54.

Snow RW, Gouws E, Omumbo J, Rapuoda B, Craig MH, Tanser FC, le Sueur D, Ouma J. (1998a) Models to predict the intensity of P. falciparum transmission: applications to the burden of disease in Kenya. *Trans R Soc Trop Med Hyg* 92:601–6.

Snow RW, Nahlen B, Palmer A, Donnelly CA, Gupta S, Marsh K. (1998b) Risk of severe malaria among African infants: direct evidence of clinical protection during early infancy. *J Infect Dis* 177: 819–822.

Snow RW, Peshu N, Forster D, Bomu G, Mitsanze E, Ngumbao E, Chisengwa R, Schellenberg JR, Hayes RJ, Newbold CI, Marsh K. (1998c) Environmental and entomological risk factors for the development of clinical malaria among children on the Kenyan coast. *Trans R Soc Trop Med Hyg* 92:381–5.

Soper HE. (1929) Interpretation of periodicity in disease-prevalence. *J.R. Statist. Soc.* 92:34–73.

StataCorp (2004) *Stata Statistical Software: Release 8.0* Collage Station Texas Stata Corporation.

Steketee RW, Nahlen BL, Parise ME, Menendez C. (2001) The burden of malaria in pregnancy in malaria-endemic areas. *Am J Trop Med Hyg* 64 (1–2 Suppl):28–35.

Takken W, Klowden MJ, Chambers GM. (1998) Effect of body size on host seeking and blood meal utilization in Anopheles gambiae sensu stricto (Diptera: Culicidae): the disadvantage of being small. *J Med Entomol* 35:639–645.

Takken W. (2002) Do insecticide-treated bednets have an effect on malaria vectors? *Trop Med Int Health* 7:1022–30.

Taylor TE. (2000) In: *Hunter's Tropical Medicine and Emerging Infectious Diseases* 8th Edition.

Teklehaimanot HD, Lipsitch M, Teklehaimanot A, Schwartz J. (2004) Weather-based prediction of P. falciparum malaria in epidemic-prone regions of Ethiopia I. Patterns of lagged weather effects reflect biological mechanisms. *Malar J* 3:41.

Thomas CJ, Lindsay SW. (2000) Local-scale variation in malaria infection amongst rural Gambian children estimated by satellite remote sensing. *Trans R Soc Trop Med Hyg.* 94:159–63.

Thomson MC, Connor SJ, Milligan PJ, Flesse SP. (1997) Mapping malaria risk in Africa: What can satellite data contribute? *Parasitolo Today* 13:313–318.

Thomson MC, Connor SJ, D'Alessandro U, Rowlingson B, Diggle P, Cresswell M, Greenwood B. (1999) Predicting malaria infection in Gambian children from satellite data and bed net use surveys: the importance of spatial correlation in the interpretation of results. *Am J Trop Med Hyg* 61:2–8.

Traoré C. (2003) Epidemiology of malaria in a holo-endemic area of rural Burkina Faso. In PhD Thesis University of Heidelberg.

Trapé JF, Lefebvre-Zante E, Legros F, Ndiaye G, Bouganali H, Druilhe P, Salem G. (1992) Vector density gradients and the epidemiology of urban malaria in Dakar, Senegal. *Am J Trop Med Hyg* 47:181–9.

Trapé J. (2001) The public health impact of chloroquine resistance in Africa. *Am J Trop Med Hyg* 64: 12–17.

Trigg PI, and Kondrachine AV. (1998a) The current global malaria situation. In: Sherman, J.W.editor. *Malaria: Parasite biology, pathogenesis and protection.* Washington D. C.: ASM Press. pp. 11–24.

Trigg PI, Kondrachine AV. (1998b) Commentary: malaria control in the 1990s. *Bull World Health Organ* 76:11–6.

Utzinger J, Tozan Y, Singer BH. (2001) Efficacy and cost-effectiveness of environmental management for malaria control. *Trop Med Int Health* 6: 677–687.

Uzochukwu BS, Onwujekwe OE. (2004) Socio-economic differences and health seeking behaviour for the diagnosis and treatment of malaria: a case study of four local government areas operating the Bamako initiative programme in south-east Nigeria. *Int J Equity Health* 3:6.

Van der Hoek W, Konradsen F, Amerasinghe PH, Perera D, Piyaratne MK, Amerasinghe FP. (2003) Towards a risk map of malaria for Sri Lanka: the importance of house location relative to vector breeding sites. *Int J Epidemiol.* 32:280–285.

Wanji S, Tanke T, Atanga SN, Ajonina C, Nicholas T, Fontenille D. (2003) Anopheles species of the mount Cameroon region: biting habits, feeding behaviour and entomological inoculation rates. *Trop Med Int Health* 8:643–9.

WHO (1993) *Implementation of the global malaria control strategy. Report of the WHO study group on the implementation of the global plan for action for malaria control 1993–2000*, WHO Technical Report Series 839, WHO, Geneva.

WHO (1997). World malaria situation in 1994. Part I. Population at risk *Wkly Epidemiol Rec.* 72:269:74.

WHO (1998) *Making a Difference in Your Life*, WHO/INF 99.1, Geneva.

WHO (1999) *The World Health Report 1999: Making a difference.* World Health Organization Geneva.

WHO (2002) *Report 2002: Reducing Risks, Promoting Healthy Life*. World Health Organization Geneva.

WHO/UNICEF (2003) *Africa Malaria Report 2003.* World Health Organization, Geneva.

Wurthwein R, Gbangou A, Sauerborn R, Schmidt CM. (2001) Measuring the local burden of disease. A study of years of life lost in sub-Saharan Africa. *Int J Epidemiol* 30:501–8.

Yé Y, Sanou A, Gbangou A, Kouyaté B. (2001) *INDEPTH. Demography and Health in Developing Countries. Volume 1*. Population, Health and Survival at INDEPTH Sites. Chapter 19 Nouna DSS. IDRC Canada.

Zhou G, Minakawa N, Githeko AK, Yan G. (2005) Climate variability and malaria epidemics in the highlands of East Africa. *Trends Parasitol* 21:54–6.

Annexes

Annex 1 The Garki Model Mathematical Equations

$$\Delta x_1 = \delta + y_2 R_1(h) - (h + \delta) x_1$$

$$\Delta x_2 = h x_1 - (1 - \delta)^N + h(t - N) x_1 (t - N) - \delta x_2$$

$$\Delta x_3 = y_3 R_2(h) - (h + \delta) x_3$$

$$\Delta x_4 = h x_3 - (1 - \delta)^N + h(t - N) x_3 (t - N) - \delta x_4$$

$$\Delta y_1 = (1 - \delta)^N + h(t - N) x_1 (t - N) - (\alpha_1 + \delta) y_1$$

$$\Delta y_2 = \alpha_1 y_1 - (\alpha_2 + R_1(h) + \delta) y_2$$

$$\Delta y_3 = \alpha_2 y_2 - (1 - \delta)^N + h(t - N) x_3 (t - N) - (R_2(h) + \delta) y_3$$

Annex 2 Informed Consent Forms for Parasitological Survey

Formulaire consentement des parents : enquête parasitologique

«Intégration des facteurs environnementaux dans la modélisation de la transmission du paludisme chez les enfants de moins de cinq ans en milieu rural au Burkina Faso»

Nom de l'enfant : ________________________ ID individuel /__/__/__/./__/__/__/-/__/__/__/
ID Ménage /__/__/./__/__/__/-/__/ Nom du chef de Ménage: ________________________

Présentation
Nous sommes du Centre de Recherche en Santé de Nouna et nous travaillons en collaboration avec le District Sanitaire. Noms et Prénom (s) et titres (Enquêteurs, Superviseurs, ...).

Cause de la rencontre
Nous voulons vous parler d'une étude qui concerne les enfants. Nous voulons savoir si vous aimeriez que vos enfants soient dans l'étude.
Pourquoi votre enfant ?
Nous avons choisi votre enfant parce que son âge est inférieur à 5 ans. Le choix a été fait au hasard.
Pourquoi cette étude ?
Nous voulons déterminer les effets des facteurs écologiques sur la transmission du paludisme. Cela nous aiderait à savoir où et quand le paludisme attaquera intensément les enfants.Sachant cela, le district sanitaire pourra prendre les mesures nécessaires pour prévenir contre le paludisme.
Comment travaillons-nous avec les enfants ?
Si vous décidez que votre enfant participe, nous lui rendrons visite chaque semaine et nous prendrons sa température (sous l'aisselle). S'il a la fièvre, nous allons faire un prélèvement de sang à partir du doigt. Nous allons analyser son sang pour voir s'il est infecté par les parasites du paludisme. Mais au début et à la fin de l'étude, nous allons faire un prélèvement de sang chez tous les enfants pour savoir s'ils ne font pas de fièvre.
Y aura-t-il des blessures ?
L'enfant ressentira une petite douleur au moment de la prise de sang, mais elle passera. La procédure que nous utilisons est sûre parce que nous utiliserons une un matériel à usage unique stérilisé.
Avantages pour l'enfant ?
Durant l'étude, si votre enfant fait la fièvre, nous lui donnerons de la chloroquine pour le traiter du paludisme Nous lui rendrons visite après deux jours. S'il ne va pas bien toujours, nous l'amènerons à la formation sanitaire et nous prendrons tous les frais en charge.
Anonymat de votre enfant ?
Nous ne dirons à personne que nous avons fait un prélèvement de sang à votre enfant. Seule l'équipe ici saura.
Obligation de participer à l'étude ?
Personne ne sera fâché ou ne vous dérangera si vous ne voulez pas que votre enfant participe à l'étude. Vous n'avez qu'à nous dire tout juste si vous voulez que votre enfant participe ou pas. Sachez que même au cours de l'étude vous avez la possibilité de retirer l'enfant.
Avez-vous des questions ?
Vous pouvez poser des questions à tout moment.

____

J'ai lu et compris ce formulaire de consentement et m'engage à laisser mon enfant participer à cette étude.
Nom du père et signature du père: ____
Date: /__/__/./__/__/./__/__/
Nom et signature du principal investigateur : ________________________________
Date: /__/__/./__/__/./__/__/

Annex 3 Cross-sectional Survey Questionnaire

L'etude" Intrégration des facteurs environnementaux dans la modélisation de la transmission du paludisme chez les enfants de moins de cinq ans en milieu rural au Burkina Faso"

Fiche enquête transversale paludologie de l'enfant n° ☐ Page 1 de 1

Medecin Nom: ☐ Code: ☐☐☐ Date: ☐☐/☐☐/☐☐
Prenom ☐

1. Indentification de l'enfant L'enfant est-il présent? (OUI, NON) ☐☐☐

Village: Menage: Chef ménage: IDCHM:

Nom et prénom de l'enfant: IDEnfant: Sexe:
DatNaiss non corrigée: DatNaiss. corrigée: Age au 13/11/03: mois
Nom et prénom de a mère: ID de la mère:

2. Interrogatoire

L'enfant a t-il eu la fièvre au cours des deux derniers jours? (OUI, NON, NSP) ☐☐☐
Si oui, l'épisode de fièvre a t-il été traité avec la chloroquine à domicile (OUI, NON, NSP) ☐☐☐
Si oui, l'épisode de fièvre a t-il été traité dans une formation sanitaire (OUI, NON, NSP) ☐☐☐
L'enfant a est-il présentement malade? (OUI, NON, NSP) ☐☐☐

3. Examen clinique

Poids en Kg	Temperature axillaire °C	Prélèvement		Score de Hackett	Autre signes cliniques
		Oui/Non/Ref	ID lame		
☐☐,☐	☐☐,☐				

4. Diagnostique clinique

____
____
____

5. Traitement reçu

____
____
____

6. Examens de laboratoire

Espèce plasmodiale	Stade parasitaire	Densité parasitaire
falciparum		
malariae		
ovale		

Annex 4 Parasitological Survey Program

Intégration des Facteurs Environnementaux dans la modélisation de la transmission du paludisme chez les enfants de moins de cinq ans en milieu rural au Burkina Faso

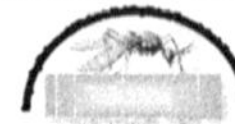

Calendrier des enquêtes paludologiques, du 1/12/03 au 30/11/04

Village____________________ Enquêteur____________________________

Année	Mois	N° sem.	Date début	Date début	Enquête paludo	Realisée
2003	Décembre	1	01/12/2003	03/12/2003	Enfant et Ménage	
		2	08/12/2003	10/12/2003	Enfant	
		3	15/12/2003	17/12/2003	Enfant	
		4	22/12/2003	24/12/2003	Enfant	
		5	29/12/2003	31/12/2003	Enfant	
2004	Janvier	6	05/01/2004	07/01/2004	Enfant et Ménage	
		7	12/01/2004	14/01/2004	Enfant	
		8	19/01/2004	21/01/2004	Enfant	
		9	26/01/2004	28/01/2004	Enfant	
	Février	10	02/02/2004	04/02/2004	Enfant et Ménage	
		11	09/02/2004	11/02/2004	Enfant	
		12	16/02/2004	18/02/2004	Enfant	
		13	23/02/2004	25/02/2004	Enfant	
	Mars	14	01/03/2004	03/03/2004	Enfant et Ménage	
		15	08/03/2004	10/03/2004	Enfant	
		16	15/03/2004	17/03/2004	Enfant	
		17	22/03/2004	24/03/2004	Enfant	
		18	29/03/2004	31/03/2004	Enfant	
	Avril	19	05/04/2004	07/04/2004	Enfant et Ménage	
		20	12/04/2004	14/04/2004	Enfant	
		21	19/04/2004	21/04/2004	Enfant	
		22	26/04/2004	28/04/2004	Enfant	
	Mai	23	03/05/2004	05/05/2004	Enfant et Ménage	
		24	10/05/2004	12/05/2004	Enfant	
		25	17/05/2004	19/05/2004	Enfant	
		26	24/05/2004	26/05/2004	Enfant	
		27	31/05/2004	02/06/2004	Enfant	
	Juin	28	07/06/2004	09/06/2004	Enfant et Ménage	
		29	14/06/2004	16/06/2004	Enfant	
		30	21/06/2004	23/06/2004	Enfant	
		31	28/06/2004	30/06/2004	Enfant	
	Juillet	32	05/07/2004	07/07/2004	Enfant et Ménage	
		33	12/07/2004	14/07/2004	Enfant	
		34	19/07/2004	21/07/2004	Enfant	
		35	26/07/2004	28/07/2004	Enfant	
	Aout	36	02/08/2004	04/08/2004	Enfant et Ménage	
		37	09/08/2004	11/08/2004	Enfant	
		38	16/08/2004	18/08/2004	Enfant	
		39	23/08/2004	25/08/2004	Enfant	
		40	30/08/2004	01/09/2004	Enfant	
	Septembre	41	06/09/2004	08/09/2004	Enfant et Ménage	
		42	13/09/2004	15/09/2004	Enfant	
		43	20/09/2004	22/09/2004	Enfant	
		44	27/09/2004	29/09/2004	Enfant	
	Octobre	45	04/10/2004	06/10/2004	Enfant et Ménage	
		46	11/10/2004	13/10/2004	Enfant	
		47	18/10/2004	20/10/2004	Enfant	
		48	25/10/2004	27/10/2004	Enfant	
	Novembre	49	01/11/2004	03/11/2004	Enfant et Ménage	
		50	08/11/2004	10/11/2004	Enfant	
		51	15/11/2004	17/11/2004	Enfant	
		52	22/11/2004	24/11/2004	Enfant	
		53	29/11/2004	01/12/2004	Enfant	

Annex 5 Parasitological Survey: Weekly Visit Form

L'etude" Intrégration des facteurs environnementaux dans la modélisation de la transmission du paludisme chez les enfants de moins de cinq ans en milieu rural au Burkina Faso"

Fiche hebdomadaire de suivie parasitologique de l'enfant

Page 1 de 2

Enquêteur Nom: Prenom: Code:

1. Indentification de l'enfant

Village Menage: Chef ménage: IDCHM:

Coordonnés GPS du menage: Latitude: Longitude:

Nom et prénom de l'enfant: IDEnfant: Sexe:

DatNaiss non corrigée: DatNaiss. corrigée: Age au 13/11/03: mois

Nom et prénom de a mère: ID de la mère:

2. Visit de l'enfant

Visite N°	Date de visite	Présent Oui/Non/Ref	Temperature axillaire °C	Prélèvement		Traitement Oui/Non/Ref	** Moustiquaire	Sign. Superv.
				Oui/Non/Ref	ID lame *			
01								
02								
03								
04								
05								
06								
07								
08								
09								
10								
11								
12								
13								
14								
15								
16								
17								
18								

* *L'identification des lames doit être composée du n° de visite et des six derniers chiffres de l'ID de l'enfant.*

** *Demandez si l'enfant a dormis sous une moustiquaire la semaine passé. Si Non, écirvez Non, si OUI demandez le type de moustiquaire Imprègnée(IMP) ou non imprègnée (NIM) et écrivez le code correspondant.*

Annex 6 Parasitological Survey: Participant Absence Form

L'etude" Intrégration des facteurs environnementaux dans la modélisation de la transmission du paludisme chez les enfants de moins de cinq ans en milieu rural au Burkina Faso"

Fiche absence

Page 1 de 1

Remplissez cette fiche pour toute absence de plus de trois jours

Enquêteur Nom: Prenom: Code:

1. Indentification de l'enfant

Village

Menage:

Chef ménage:

IDCHM:

Nom et prénom de l'enfant:

IDEnfant:

Sexe:

Nom et prénom de a mère:

IDMère:

2. Absences

Remplissez le tableau ci-dessous pour chaque absence constatée. Chaque ligne represente un épisode d'absence

N° Absence	Date du constat	Destination *	Va t-il/elle revenir, Oui/Non/NSP	Date probable de retour	Date Effective de retour	Nbr de jr abs
01						
02						
03						
04						
05						
06						

* *Pour la destination utilisez les codes suivants: CIS=village de cissé, KOD= village de Kodougou, GON=village de Goni, NOU, Village de Nouna, VIN=Autre village du DSS, CHP=Champ, NSP= Ne sait pas*

Annex 7 Parasitological Survey: Treatment Form

L'etude" Intrégration des facteurs environnementaux dans la modélisation de la transmission du paludisme chez les enfants de moins de cinq anx en milieu rural au Burkina Faso"

Fiche de traitement des enfants, épisodes fébriles Page 1 de 1

Enquêteur Nom: Prenom: Code:

1. Indentification de l'enfant

Village: Menage: Chef ménage: IDCHM:

Nom et prénom de l'enfant: IDEnfant: Sexe:

DatNaiss non corrigée: DatNaiss. corrigée: Age au 13/11/03: mois

Nom et prénom de a mère: ID de la mère:

2. Traitement

Cette fiche est à remplir chaque fois qu'un enfat fait la fièvre et que vous lui administrez un traitement

Si la température mesurée est comprise entre 37,5 et 38,5°c, donner de la chroroquine seule

Si la température mesurée est supérieure ou égale à 38,6°c, donner de la chloroquine et du paracétamol

Dans tous les cas continuez la chloroquine pendant 3 jours successifs

En présence de signes de complications (vomissement, déshydratation, ictère, convulsions, coma...) aider les parents à amener l'enfant au CSPS

Numéro de la visite

Jour	Date de visite	Présent Oui/Non/Ref	Temperature axillaire °C	Chloroquine		Paracétamol		Observations
				Oui/Non	Dose	Oui/Non	Dose et nbr de prise	
01			,					
02			,					
02			,					

Annex 8 Parasitological Survey: Laboratories Results Form

L'etude" Intrégration des facteurs environnementaux dans la modélisation de la transmission du paludisme chez les enfants de moins de cinq ans en milieu rural au Burkina Faso"

Fiche de laboratoire de l'enfant

Page 1 de 1

Laboratoire

1. Indentification de l'enfant

Village: Menage: Chef ménage: IDCHM:

Nom et prénom de l'enfant: IDEnfant: Sexe:

DatNaiss non corrigée: DatNaiss. corrigée: Age au 13/11/03: mois

Nom et prénom de a mère: ID de la mère:

2. Analyse

Prèlevement	**Parasite**			
	Stade	***Plasmodium falciparum***	***Plasmodium malaria***	***Plasmodium ovale***
Date:	1:			
ID lame:	Densité			
	2:			
Nom laborantin:	Densité			
	3:			
	Densité			
Date:	1:			
ID lame:	Densité			
	2:			
Nom laborantin:	Densité			
	3:			
	Densité			
Date:	1:			
ID lame:	Densité			
	2:			
Nom laborantin:	Densité			
	3:			
	Densité			

Annex 9 Household Survey Forms

L'etude" Intrégration des facteurs environnementaux dans la modélisation de la transmission du paludisme chez les enfants de moins de cinq ans en milieu rural au Burkina Faso"

Date de visite

Fiche mensuelle du ménage Mois_______________

Enquêteur: Nom: Prenom: Code

Village Menage: Chef ménage: IDCHM:

Coordonnés GPS du menage: Latitude: Longitude:

1. Historique du paludisme dans le ménage

Demandez pour chaque membre du ménage s'il a été malade du paludisme les 30 derniers jours precédent votre passage et remplissez le tableau ci -dessous

Membres	Sexe	Age	A t-il eu le palu? OUI=oui NON=Non NSP=Sait pas	A t-il pris un antipalu? OUI=oui, NON=Non NSP=Sait pas	Quel antipalu? CHL=Chloroquine FAN=Fansidar TRA=Traditionnel AUT:Autre	Dose	
						Comp/jour	Nbr jour

2. Utilisation de moustiquaire

a) Avez-vous un ou des moustiquaires dans votre ménage ? *(Oui=OUI, Non=NON)*

b) Si oui combien de moustiquaires au total *(99 pour non applicable)*

Nombre de moustiquaires non-imprègnées *(99 pour non applicable)*

Nombre de moustiquaires imprègnées *(99 pour non applicable)*

c) Ces moustiquaires sont-elles utilisées par des membres de votre ménage *(Oui=OUI, Non=NON, Non applicable=NAP)*

3. Ménage et son environnent (30 mètre aux alentours)

a) Type de maison (considerez surtout là où dort l'enfant)

Mur *(Banco= BAN, Dur=DUR, Semi-dur=SDU)*

Toit *(Banco= BAN, Tole=TOL, Paille=PAI, Tuile=TUI*

b) Y a t-il au moins un point d'eau dans un rayon de 30 mètres autour du ménage *(Oui=OUI, Non=NON)*

c) Y a t-il au des champs(cultures) dans un rayon de 30 mètres autour du ménage *(Oui=OUI, Non=NON)*

d) Y a t-il au des enclos d'animaux dans un rayon de 30 mètres autour du ménage *(Oui=OUI, Non=NON)*

e) Quelle est la distance du ménage à une gîte larvaire potentielle? *mètres*

Superviseur: *Nom et prénoms:* *Date:*

Signature:

Annex 10 Entomological Survey: Mosquitoes Capture Program

Intégration des Facteurs Environnementaux dans la modélisation de la transmission du paludisme chez les enfants de moins de cinq ans en milieu rural

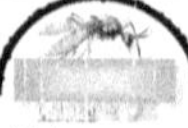

Calendrier de capture des moustiques, du 1/12/03 au 30/11/04

Date Cpt	Goni *IDMenage*	Cissé *IDMenage*	Kodougou *IDMenage*	Nouna *IDMenage*	Type LTC, HLC, PS
01/12/2003	17294A0	837A0	2017A0	42304A1	LTC
02/12/2003	17488A0	811A0	2050B0	42231A4	LTC
	17438A0	852A0	2018A0	42141A3	LTC
	17133A0	833A0	20151A0	42269A4	LTC
01/01/2004	17315A0	86A0	20113A0	42339B5	LTC, HLC
02/01/2004	17100B0	82A0	20142B0	42155A4	LTC, HLC
	17109A0	868B0	20132A0	42102A4	LTC, HLC
	17322A0	839A0	20180A0	42228A2	LTC, HLC
01/02/2004	172A0	202A0	20189A0	4220A4	LTC
02/02/2004	17326A0	838A0	20122B0	42172A3	LTC
	17329A	873A0	2027A0	428A1	LTC
	17324A0	851A0	20173A0	42292A4	LTC
01/03/2004	17256A0	862A0	2079B0	4277A2	LTC, HLC
02/03/2004	17305A0	816A0	20101A0	4298A4	LTC, HLC
	17246A0	863A0	20238A0	4261A5	LTC, HLC
	17301B0	853A0	20128A0	42218A5	LTC, HLC
01/04/2004	17288A0	856A0	20121A0	4278A5	LTC
02/04/2004	17299A0	819A0	20235A0	42356A5	LTC
	17302A0	849A0	20126A0	42183A1	LTC
	17242A0	848A0	2038A0	42117A4	LTC
01/05/2004	17257A0	838B0	2028A0	42218B2	LTC, HLC
02/05/2004	17529A0	816B0	20171A0	42100A1	LTC, HLC
	17293B0	853B0	20140A0	42410A1	LTC, HLC
	17285A0	855A0	20134B0	42285A4	LTC, HLC
01/06/2004	179A0	847A0	20152A0	4264A3	LTC,PS
02/06/2004	1783A0	835A0	20102A0	42141A5	LTC
	17284A0	813A0	2031A0	4249A1	LTC
	17276A0	8111A0	2023A0	4216A2	LTC
01/07/2003	17269A0	830E 0	2025A0	4228A4	LTC, HLC
02/07/2003	17310A0	20142A0	2030A0	42160B4	LTC, HLC
	17138A0	830D0	20237A0	42124B2	LTC, HLC
	17536A0	828A0	20247A0	4268A2	LTC, HLC
01/08/2004	1777A0	85A0	20145A0	4273A5	LTC, HLC,PS
02/08/2004	17227B0	861A0	20236A0	42218A2	LTC, HLC
	17527A0	841A0	20149A0	42187B2	LTC, HLC
	17506A0	864A0	20192B0	42297C4	LTC, HLC
01/09/2004	17494A0	815A0	20194A0	42292A4	LTC, HLC
02/09/2004	17504A0	818A0	2097A0	42204A5	LTC, HLC
	1752A0	854A0	2097A0	4218A1	LTC, HLC
	1776A0	866A0	2096B0	42160B4	LTC, HLC
01/10/2004	1760A0	865A0	20122C0	42428A5	LTC, HLC,PS
02/10/2004	17524A0	8112A0	20195A0	42102A4	LTC, HLC
	1764A0	8114A0	2011A0	42438A4	LTC, HLC
	1765A0	813B0	2022A0	42124A3	LTC, HLC
01/11/2004	17441A0	821A0	2012A0	42455A4	LTC
02/11/2004	1761A0	8108A0	20225A0	4241A2	LTC
	1762A0	820D0	20100A0	4228A4	LTC
	17596A0	826A0	20226a0	42348A3	LTC

Annex 11 Entomological Survey: Human Land Trap Forms

Intégration des Facteurs Environnementaux dans la modélisation de la transmission du paludisme chez les enfants de moins de cinq ans en milieu rural au Burkina Faso

Fiche de relevé de capture HLC

Capture: interieure I__I Exterieure I__I

Village:________________ Mois:___________

Cod ménage:I__I__I__I I__I I__I

Date (J1) : **Heures Début :** **Heure fin :**

Genre		Anopheles					Mans		Aedes				Culex					
Heures	Ag	Af	An	Ac	Autre		Mu	Ma	Aa	Af			Cq	Cp				Autre
18-19																		
19-20																		
20-21																		
21-22																		
22-23																		
23-24																		
24-01																		
01-02																		
02-03																		
03-04																		
04-05																		
05-06																		
Total																		

Date (J2) : **Heures Début :** **Heure fin :**

Genre		Anopheles					Mans		Aedes				Culex					
Heures	Ag	Af	An	Ac	Autre		Mu	Ma	Aa	Af			Cq	Cp				Autre
18-19																		
19-20																		
20-21																		
21-22																		
22-23																		
23-24																		
24-01																		
01-02																		
02-03																		
03-04																		
04-05																		
05-06																		
Total																		

Total J1+J2 Captures

Genre		Anopheles					Mans		Aedes				Culex					
Heures	Ag	Af	An	Ac	Autre		Mu	Ma	Aa	Af			Cq	Cp				Autre
18-19																		
19-20																		
20-21																		
21-22																		
22-23																		
23-24																		
24-01																		
01-02																		
02-03																		
03-04																		
04-05																		
05-06																		
Total																		

Annex 12 Entomological Survey: Light Trap Capture Form

Etude: «Intégration des Facteurs Environnementaux dans la modélisation de la transmission du paludisme chez les enfants de moins de cinq ans en milieu rural au Burkina Faso»

Fiche de capture LTC

Agent de captures

Noms et prénoms	Code

Identification du point de capture		Identificatio	
Village:		Nom, Prénom:	
IDMenage:	I I I I.I I.I I	Sexe:	Mas ❑ Fem ❑
Nombre de personnes dans la maison:	I I I	Date naissance:	I I I.I I I.I I I
Nombre d'enfant de moins de cinq:	I I I		

Autres personnes dormant sous la moustiquaire :Non❑

Si oui, remplissez le tableau ci-dessous:

Noms et prénoms	Age	Sexe

Type de protection individuelle

Présence de moustiquaires	Oui ❑ Non ❑
Si oui, type	Imprégnée ❑
Nombre de personne protégées	I I I
Présence d'autres	Oui ❑ Non ❑
Pulvérisations domestiques (insecticides):	Oui ❑ Non ❑
Si oui, date dernière pulvérisation	I I I.I I I.I I I
Utilisation de répulsifs (Mosquito, répulsifs pharmaceutiques)	Oui ❑ Non ❑

Fonctionnement du piège

Heure	Date J1 :	Date J2 :	Observation
Piège en marche à 21h	Oui ❑ Non ❑	Oui ❑ Non ❑	
Piège en marche à 6h	Oui ❑ Non ❑	Oui ❑ Non ❑	

Observation

Pluie seule	Oui ❑ Non ❑	Heure :
Grand vent seul	Oui ❑ Non ❑	Heure :
Grand vent et pluie	Oui ❑ Non ❑	Heure :

Présence des animaux domestiques

Désignation	Présence	Dans la cour	Dans la maison
Bœufs/Veaux	Oui ❑ Non ❑		
Anes/Chevaux	Oui ❑ Non ❑		
Chèvres/Moutons	Oui ❑ Non ❑		
Chiens/Chats	Oui ❑ Non ❑		
Porcs	Oui ❑ Non ❑		
Oiseaux	Oui ❑ Non ❑		
Autres (spécifier)	Oui ❑ Non ❑		

Annex 12 *Continued*

Fiche de détermination des espèces de moustiques

Jour 2 Dates : I__I__I.I__I__I.I__I__I Heure début:______fin:_______

Espèces	Femelles						
	A jeun	*Partial gorgée*	*Gorgées*	*Semi-gravides*	*Sub-gr et gravides*	**Total**	**Males**
An. gambiae							
An.funestus							
C.quinquefasciatus							
Mansonia							
Total							

Jour 2 Dates : I__I__I.I__I__I.I__I__I Heure début:______fin:_______

Espèces	Femelles						
	A jeun	*Partial gorgée*	*Gorgées*	*Semi-gravides*	*Sub-gr et gravides*	**Total**	**Males**
An. gambiae							
An.funestus							
C.quinquefasciatus							
Mansonia							
Total							

Total : Jour 1 + Jour 2

Espèces	Femelles						
	A jeun	*Partial gorgée*	*Gorgées*	*Semi-gravides*	*Sub-gr et gravides*	**Total**	**Males**
An. gambiae							
An.funestus							
C.quinquefasciatus							
Mansonia							
Total							

Annex 13 Entomological Survey: Pyrethrum Spray Capture Form

Fiche de récolte et examen adultes

Pour capture au pyrèthre, capture manuelles te piège a sorties

Type de récolte

CP
CM
PS

Village ____________
Date de récolte ____________
Concession ____________
Maison ____________
Type de maison ____________
Récolte commencée ____________
Récolte arrêtée ____________

Nom(s) de(s) captureur(s)
____
____

Espèces	Femelles						Males
	A jeun	Partial gorgées	Gorgées	Semi gravides	Sub-gr et gravides	Total	
Anophèles gambiae							
Anophèles funestus							
Anophèles nili							
Culex sp							
Mansonia sp							

Nombre total de personnes :			
Nombre d'enfants (,10ans)			
Nombre de fenêtres			
Nombre de draps utilisés			Si CP
Type d'insecticide utilisé			
Position du piège a sortie	Fenêtre	Porte	Si PS
Exposition de la fenêtre/porte	nord	est	
	ouest	sud	

Présence de moustiquaires	Oui	Non
Nombre de personnes protéges		
Utilisation de serpentins/insecticide	Oui	Non
Présence de feu pendant la nuit	Oui	Non

Présence des animaux domestiques		Cours	Maison
Bœuf/Veaux	Non		
Anes/chevaux	Non		
Chèvres/montons	Non		
Chiens/Chats	Non		
Porcs	Non		
Oiseaux (poulet, canards..)	Non		
Autres (spécifier)	Non		

Annex 14 Entomological Survey: Mosquitoes Dissection Form

FICHE DE DISSECTION ANOPHELES

Lieu: **Mois:** **Observation:**

N°	Date	Menage	Case	Ext.(0)	CSH	H	Espece	Etat de Repletion					Ovaire			Echan	Salivaire	
				Int.(0)	CFR			Aj	1/2Gg	Gr	1/2Gr	Gr	Diss	N	P	tillon	Elisa	
1																		
2																		
3																		
4																		
5																		
6																		
7																		
8																		
9																		
10																		
11																		
12																		
13																		
14																		
15																		
16																		
17																		
18																		
19																		
20																		
21																		
22																		
23																		
24																		
25																		
26																		
27																		
28																		
29																		

Index

For Product Safety Concerns and Information please contact our EU
representative GPSR@taylorandfrancis.com
Taylor & Francis Verlag GmbH, Kaufingerstraße 24, 80331 München, Germany

www.ingramcontent.com/pod-product-compliance
Lightning Source LLC
Chambersburg PA
CBHW070728220326
41598CB00024BA/3346
9781138619579